DIABETES
The GlŭcograF® method for normalizing blood sugar

DIABETES
The GlucograF® method for normalizing blood sugar

Richard K. Bernstein, M.D.

JEREMY P. TARCHER, INC.
Los Angeles
Distributed by Houghton Mifflin Company
Boston

Library of Congress Cataloging in Publication Data

Bernstein, Richard K.
  Diabetes: the GlucograF® method for normalizing blood sugar.

  Includes index.
  1. Insulin. 2. Diabetes—Treatment. 3. Blood sugar—Analysis. 4. Patient
monitoring. 5. Self medication. I. Diabetes Research & Training Center of
the Albert Einstein College of Medicine & Montefiore Hospital & Medical
Center. II. Title.
RC661.I6B47 1984   616.4'62061   83-24257
ISBN 0-87477-314-8

Originally published by Crown Publishers, Inc., in 1981.

Jeremy P. Tarcher, Inc.
9110 Sunset Blvd.
Los Angeles, CA 90069

GlucograF® is a trademark of Richard K. Bernstein.

Manufactured in the United States of America
V 10 9 8 7 6 5 4 3 2 1

To my family and the families of diabetics everywhere
Patienta brevis amor longus

and

To the memory of Samuel M. Rosen, M.D.

A, 4 - 5,6

CONTENTS

PREFACE TO THE NEW EDITION

PLEASE READ THIS PREFACE. It contains several new "tips" for facilitating blood sugar control that do not appear farther on in the text. For maximum comprehension, read it again after finishing the book.

Since the publication of the original hardcover edition of this book in 1981, a number of developments have occurred that warrant some discussion, although they do not change the usefulness of the contents.

One development, of course, was my graduation from medical school and completion of subsequent postgraduate training. I can honestly say that while this experience added to my understanding of the physiologic and biochemical mechanisms important to the treatment of diabetes, I've found no equally satisfactory alternative to the GlucograF method for blood glucose control.

I have had many opportunities, however, during my training and in my private medical practice to apply the dietary approach described in this book to Type II (non-insulin-dependent) diabetics and to nondiabetics with a low blood sugar condition known as "reactive hypoglycemia." In both instances our low-carbohydrate diet was very successful in stabilizing blood glucose levels. The key to this success was the prescribing of three to six daily meals or snacks (depending upon the individual) with no more than twenty grams of carbohydrate at any one time. The remaining intake at a meal consisted as much as possible of low-saturated-fat, high-protein foods. This same diet was also used to wean certain poorly controlled maturity-onset diabetics from insulin. These people responded with normal blood sugars to oral antidiabetic agents administered according to the following pattern: small to moderate doses of a long-acting medication (such as chlorpropamide) once daily,[1] and small to moderate doses of a short-acting oral agent (tolbutamide) about three hours prior to each meal. To my knowledge, this combined use of long- and short-acting drugs has not been previously reported.

During the past three years, many new products have appeared on the market for the self-monitoring of blood sugar by patients themselves. Several unsatisfactory products have been replaced by better ones, but many of the new products are also unsatisfactory. At present the marketplace is changing so rapidly that if we had reviewed each product, many would have been replaced by newer ones by the time this book was printed. With the exception of the Ames Glucometer, none of the blood glucose meters described in Chapter 8 are currently in production. We can, however, give several important guidelines to anyone purchasing reagent strips or meters for measuring blood sugar:

1. If you are a Type I diabetic (as described on page 47), do not attempt to read blood sugar strips by eye; use a meter. You need better accuracy than visual readings can give. This is also good, but not mandatory advice for those mild Type II diabetics being treated with small doses of insulin.

2. Only use those brands of blood sugar strips for which the manufacturer supplies three liquid glucose control solutions: high, normal, and low. This will permit you to check the accuracy of your technique and your materials.

3. Do not purchase a blood glucose meter until you have seen the model demonstrated with the three aforementioned glucose control solutions. The meter should read

---

1. Or an intermediate-acting oral agent (tolazamide or acetohexamide) every twelve hours.

within 15 percent of the stated value for each solution. If the stated value is a range, such as 90–110, then allow no more than a 15 percent variation from the midpoint of the range. Even with less than a 15 percent variation, users should correct their readings for each new vial of reagent strips to compensate for these variations.

In 1983, human insulin became available to patients living in the United States. It offers a few important advantages to people who want to maintain normal blood sugars:

1. Human Regular or crystalline insulin will lower blood sugar more rapidly than animal insulin. As a result, patients who previously injected forty-five minutes before mealtime may now wait until twenty-five minutes before mealtime— a great convenience.

2. A minority of Type I diabetics still experience unexplained blood sugar swings even when following the GlucograF regimen. These individuals usually have a history of skin reactions to injected insulin, allergies, hay fever, asthma, or insulin resistance during childhood. In most cases, the use of human insulin reduces or eliminates these swings, probably by curtailing the stimulation of antibodies to insulin. Unfortunately it usually takes two to three months for the transition from animal to human insulin to become effective. During this transition period blood sugar swings may become more severe.

3. Human insulin is a must for pregnant insulin users and for new insulin users who have never been treated with animal insulins. This will minimize the amount of insulin antibody production and thereby reduce the likelihood of certain known and speculated problems.[2]

Care should be taken when switching from animal to

---

2. Such as fetal insulin resistance in the case of pregnancy, difficulty with blood sugar control, deposition of immune complexes in blood vessel walls, kidneys, and other organs, etc.

human insulin. In our experience, human Regular insulin is usually about 25 percent more effective than pork insulin and perhaps 35 percent more effective than the common beef-pork mixtures. For most adult Type I patients one unit of human Regular insulin will lower blood glucose 40 mg/dl if injected subcutaneously and 45 mg/dl if injected intramuscularly.

During the past few years a number of major diabetes centers have been attempting to secure blood sugar normalization in Type I diabetics with the aid of blood glucose self-monitoring. Several researchers have observed what is now called the "dawn phenomenon" in a sizable minority of their patients. These patients exhibit sudden increases of blood glucose in the mid morning that seem to be resistant to increased evening doses of long-acting insulin. When the evening dose is raised enough to cause normal 6 A.M. blood sugars, it usually also causes hypoglycemia at about 2 A.M. A number of studies have reported attempts to find a cause for this phenomenon. As of this writing the cause is still undetermined. We've encountered our share of "dawn" patients and, while not finding the cause (we suspect it relates to the immune system), have been able to treat the condition with some degree of success using one or a combination of the following techniques:

1. Taking the evening dose of longer-acting insulin about fifteen or sixteen hours after the morning dose instead of twelve hours after the morning dose (as suggested in Chapter 12).

2. A complete switch over to human insulin—both long- and short-acting forms. Most of our experience in this respect is with human Lente insulin (Monotard in the U.S.A.) and human Regular insulin (Actrapid in the U.S.A.). Lente is actually an intermediate-acting insulin and may not last long enough for some patients. We therefore expect to

change to human Ultralente (a longer-acting form) when it becomes available.

If the nighttime dose of longer-acting insulin is 8 units or more, and morning blood sugars are still high, we ask people to split this dose into two injections. For example, two shots of 4 units each instead of one 8-unit dose. The two injections are given in different places but at the same time. This probably causes less inflammation at the injection sites with subsequent reduced destruction of insulin by certain immune factors that may be present in the skin.

3. Small to moderate doses of an intermediate-acting oral hypoglycemic agent (tolazamide or acetohexamide) at bedtime or a long-acting agent (chlorpropamide) in the middle of the day. These drugs do not directly cause blood sugar reduction in Type I patients but may somehow reduce postreceptor impairment of glucose utilization in people who have this form of insulin resistance. Thus, the oral medication is only effective at the time of day when it is actually needed and does not necessarily introduce an added risk of nocturnal hypoglycemia.

Cost of products for blood sugar measurement have also changed over the past three years, and many of the prices cited in the text are no longer valid. In particular, the prices of reagent strips have increased slightly and the costs of blood glucose meters have dropped dramatically (to about $150 in the U.S.A. and to about $100 in Canada).

In Chapter 12, entitled "The Physiologic Use of Insulin," we originally suggested mixing the long- and short-acting insulin doses in the same syringe before breakfast and dinner. This was favored in the expectation that patients would find one injection prior to each meal more benign than two injections. We pointed out, however, that the short-acting (Regular) insulin is effective in about half the time if it is not mixed with the longer-acting insulin, thus permitting less of a delay between injecting and eating. In clinical practice, it turns out that people readily adjust to multiple injections but complain about the long time delay. Since separate injections lead to more predictable blood sugars anyway, we now strongly favor this approach.

Shortly after the original printing of this book I was stunned by the sudden death of my beloved colleague Sam Rosen, M.D., who had contributed an important chapter entitled "Why Normalize Blood Glucose?" (Chapter 2). It was Sam who initially prodded me to write a "manual" to facilitate the training of his patients in this method. We had given the original draft a dry run by circulating copies to a number of patients whom we treated jointly every Sunday morning for a year while I was in medical training. The feelings of loss shared by the patients and associates of this brilliant, kindly idealist are beyond my capacity to express.

Richard K. Bernstein, M.D.
January 1984

ACKNOWLEDGMENTS

The regimen described in this manual is based upon the use of both short-acting and long-acting insulins: Regular insulin and Ultralente insulin respectively. The original regimen used by the author was based upon three daily doses of Regular insulin used jointly with intermediate-acting insulins such as Lente or NPH. It was found, however, that the time duration of these intermediate insulins was too brief for the satisfactory treatment of a large percentage of patients. The solution to this problem was proposed and tested by Sheldon Bleicher, M.D.[1] Dr. Bleicher introduced the joint use of Regular and Ultralente insulins to most of his insulin-dependent patients, at a time when virtually all such patients in the U.S. and elsewhere [2] were being treated with the intermediate insulins. Furthermore, his successful use of a *mixture* of Regular and Ultralente insulins ran counter to the printed instructions of insulin manufacturers. In addition, Dr. Bleicher was, to our knowledge, the first physician to use the regimen described in this manual in routine clinical practice. Prior thereto, he was one of the small minority of diabetologists who publicly advocated the use of Regular insulin before every meal.

The author is indebted to a number of individuals with special interests in the treatment of diabetes who were espe-

---

1. Chairman, Department of Medicine, Brooklyn–Cumberland Medical Center; Professor of Medicine, Downstate Medical Center of the State University of New York.

2. Six months prior to the first published disclosure of Bleicher's work, M. Phillips and associates at the Radcliffe Infirmary, Oxford, reported on the use of one daily dose of Ultralente plus two injections of Regular insulin before two of the three daily meals. The doses used were typically three times as great as those used by Bleicher.

cially helpful in the preparation of this manual. These include:

John A. Galloway, M.D., of Eli Lilly and Company, who
reviewed the chapters relating to insulin and its use and
made many valuable suggestions that were incorporated in
the final manuscript.

John Spratt, exercise physiologist, who made a number of
contributions to the chapter on exercise.

Jay S. Skyler, M.D., who read every word of the manuscript and spotted a number of significant typographical
errors.

Sam Seifter, Ph.D., who reviewed the manuscript and provided important corrections.

The directors of the Einstein/Montefiore Diabetes Research and Training Center, all of whom reviewed the manuscript.

Sam Rosen, M.D., who took time from a busy schedule to
research and write Chapter 2, "Why Normalize Blood Glucose?"

Judith Wylie-Rosett, Ed.D., R.D., who reviewed and corrected the chapter on diet and who was the principal source
for information used in the food lists (Appendix A).

Stephen B. Lewis, M.D.; Joel R. Poole, M.D.; James K.
Schmitt, M.D.; Arie Maman, M.D.; and Michael M. Bliziotes, M.D., whose clinical investigations resulted in their
article "Management of the Diabetic Undergoing Surgery,"
which was especially written for this manual and appears as
Appendix B.

Robert Tattersall, M.D., and Ellen Gerson both enthusiastically granted us permission to reproduce their articles
that had been printed elsewhere. These appear in Chapter 1
and as Appendix C, respectively.

Dagmar Friedman directed the author's attention to important reference material utilized in Chapters 1 and 4.

Eli Lilly and Company provided the artwork for Figure 1, and some of the information utilized in Appendix H.

We are also grateful to the following for granting permission to reproduce portions of their publications:

The American Diabetes Association *(Diabetes)*

The American Foundation for the Blind *(Journal of Visual Impairment)*

Springer-Verlag *(Diabetologia)*

Special thanks are owed to the five authors of Chapter 4, who were willing to share their personal experiences with diabetes: Ellen B. Lanners, Deborah Sloan, Dr. Paul Shevin, Clara Ducham, and J.C.

The ultimate widespread availability of this manual is due to the foresight of Marian Behrman of Crown Publishers, Inc.

PREFACE

This manual is addressed to physicians, nurses, and para-medical personnel interested in the treatment of diabetes mellitus, as well as to diabetic patients and their families. While we are concerned principally with a new treatment for insulin-dependent diabetes, some of the information set forth may also be of interest to patients who can be controlled by combinations of diet, exercise, and oral drugs.

This is not a primer for the newly diagnosed patient. A number of such introductory texts already exist and several excellent basic presentations are listed in Appendix E. Therefore, we do not cover such subjects as "how to inject insulin," "urine testing," "causes of diabetes," "what is diabetes," "use of dietary exchange lists," etc.

Because I am not yet a physician, and because the method of treatment presented here is very unconventional, it is appropriate for me to give the reader a brief history of its origin.

I am an engineer and have been diabetic for 34 years, since the age of 12½. With one exception,[1] I do not show clinical signs of any of the grave medical complications that can be found in most long-term diabetics.

During the winter of 1970–71, I experienced a period of extreme swings in daily blood sugar that lasted a number of months. Although most of my urine tests indicated the presence of considerable amounts of glucose, I was confused by symptoms of low blood sugar that were much more frequent than the occasional sugar-free urines. My natural distress and anxiety were further compounded by a change in ability to focus my eyes on distant objects that was occurring gradually

---

1. Radiographs of my legs, taken 9 years ago, show likely calcium deposits along major blood vessels. These x-rays were taken before I began to use the treatment regimen described in this manual.

over the same few months. I was certain that this related to a chronic state of low or high blood sugar, but couldn't determine which.

At about this time, as I was leafing through a clinical laboratory journal (I had been research director of a company that manufactured equipment for clinical laboratories), I stumbled upon an advertisement for a new meter that would enable laboratories to measure blood sugar levels in one minute, using one drop of blood from a finger puncture. I phoned the manufacturer and was told that these meters were not available to patients. Nevertheless, since my wife is a physician, I was able to order a meter in her name. (Fortunately, this prohibition no longer exists, and perhaps 20,000 patients throughout the world now own more modern versions of this meter supplied by at least four different manufacturers.)

With this new device, I was rapidly able to determine that my blood sugar was very high much of the time, and that my symptoms of insulin reactions were false about half the time. (This is a common problem in insulin-dependent diabetes, which is discussed elsewhere in this manual.) I raised my insulin dose, brought my blood sugars to within a more reasonable range and put the meter away in a closet. Since the disposable test strips, used with the meter, then cost 45 cents each, it made no sense to continue a costly regimen that I thought was no longer necessary.

For most of my life, I had been aware of the medical complications that eventually afflicted most diabetics. I even had nightmares about being blind or stricken with kidney disease (a common cause of death in juvenile onset diabetes). I also knew that a number of professional athletes had succeeded in living long lives with juvenile diabetes and, according to press reports, did not seem to develop the complications. So, for many years, I strenuously exercised for 1½ hours every day at a gymnasium near my office. Seven years ago (1974), however, my work load had grown to a point where I could no longer spare the long "lunch hour" that I had been spending in the gym. I decided to build a professionally equipped gym in my home.

Naturally, I expected that the Internal Revenue Service would allow me to take an income tax deduction for this valid medical expense. My accountants, however, advised me that the tax examiner would automatically challenge any large deductions, and that I'd better be prepared to justify the importance of daily exercise. They added that the letter my physician had submitted would probably be inadequate. In an attempt to get more validation, I phoned the local academy of medicine library, and ordered a computer search of the diabetes literature, covering the prior five years. For the computer, I listed the names of the more common complications and, of course, the word "exercise." I expected to be deluged with references documenting the efficacy of physical exercise in preventing these complications.

I was deluged—but not in the manner I had expected. Among dozens of computer-generated references, only two related to exercise. One tied activity levels to heart disease rates in nondiabetic London bus drivers versus fare collectors. The other article related exercise to reduction of triglyceride (fat) levels in the blood. The remaining dozens of articles added up to overwhelming evidence that, in animals, at least, the complications of diabetes were directly or indirectly attributable to *elevated blood glucose levels.*

At about this time, my wife, Anne, pointed out to me that I was spending much of my weekends either in a hypoglycemic state, entering such a state, or recovering—a process that can leave one drained of energy for many hours. I was short-tempered and not an appropriate weekend companion for my wife and three children. Furthermore, they were all concerned about the continuous hazard that frequent hypoglycemia imposed.

I had no choice. If I were to reduce the daily insulin reac-

tions (hypoglycemia) and the likelihood of the dreaded complications, I would somehow have to normalize my blood
sugar and keep it normal virtually all the time.

My first step was to take the blood glucose meter out of the
closet and put it into daily use. I started with 3 daily blood
sugar measurements, but eventually found that the information obtained was incomplete. I now measure my blood
sugar at least 6 times each day. I changed one aspect of my
regimen at a time, observing the effects on blood glucose.
Over the course of a year, my diet, use of insulin, and timing
of insulin and meals had changed so dramatically that they
bore little relation to what I had been taught or had read
regarding the treatment of diabetes. *But my blood sugars
were normal—90 percent of the time.* Where my original
daily blood sugar range was from 20 milligrams per deciliter
(very low) to over 400 mg/dl (very high), my current range is
typically 70 mg/dl to 130 mg/dl, with most values converg-
ing on 100 mg/dl.

After that first year, I observed that my chronic acne had
cleared up, fatty growths on my eyelids (xanthomas) disap-
peared, and I stopped producing kidney stones (calcium ox-
alate). Frequent skin and sinus infections no longer occurred.
I no longer felt continually tired, and now required only 5 to
6 hours sleep each night, versus the 9 hours that I seemed to
need previously. I had reduced my insulin dose from 80 units
per day to 26 units per day (now 20 units per day) and reduced serum cholesterol and triglyceride values (commonly
elevated in diabetics) to as low as 130 mg/dl and 29 mg/dl
respectively.[2] The frequency and severity of insulin reactions (hypoglycemia) dropped considerably, and as a result,
the emotional stress that diabetes had continually forced on
our family was eased. My life style became less restricted
because the rigid timing of meals and snacks formerly re-

---

2. Recent values of glycosylated hemoglobin (HbA_{1c}) and high density
lipoproteins are 4 percent and 89 mg/dl, respectively.

quired to offset the effects of large doses of intermediate-acting insulin was no longer necessary. My chronic gray pallor vanished, and for the first time in 27 years I started to look healthy. Suddenly, at age 40, I began to develop a physique. Years of exercising, with elevated blood sugar levels, did little for muscular development, but a few months of the same exercise at normal blood sugars had clearly visible results. The continuous hunger that I had experienced for so many years faded away as blood sugar control improved. I was, therefore, no longer tempted into random snacking and could even skip entire meals without discomfort.

Of great importance to me was the belief that I was probably protecting myself from the constant threat of the crippling complications. Furthermore, I felt that I was in control of that part of my physiology (blood sugar) which had so cruelly frustrated me for so many years. The investment of less than 20 minutes per day in controlling my diabetes was truly paying off across the board.

After contemplating my new life for a few months, I started to think about the millions of insulin-dependent diabetics who were still living in the prison from which I had escaped. I've spent much of the past seven years attempting to familiarize clinicians and researchers around the world with this method for achieving physiologically normal blood sugar. It is now being used successfully by many diabetics. Clearly, my own success was not unique. The emotional freedom that results, was to my amazement common to others.

Although medical journals have published elements of the new regimen, it has not appeared in a complete step-by-step guide that can be followed jointly by both patient and physician. This manual is a response to repeated requests by clinicians for such a guide.

With modern technology and medical science advancing at an accelerating pace, it is reasonable to expect that other techniques, also capable of normalizing blood glucose, will eventually become available to patients. In order to avoid confusion between our regimen and possible alternate future regimens, we have coined the term "GLUCOGRAF method" and will use it to designate the particular combination of techniques that is utilized in this manual.

The GLUCOGRAF manual is intended to serve as an operating manual for physicians, and simultaneously as a training manual that the clinician can dispense to diabetic patients. Most of the chapters begin with a simplified summary of major points. This will hopefully facilitate rapid review after the initial reading. Technical terms are defined for lay readers throughout the text and again in a glossary at the end of the manual.

An early draft of this manual has been used by certain physicians and patients at the Einstein/Montefiore Diabetes Research and Training Center of the Albert Einstein College of Medicine for up to 1½ years prior to publication. I feel that we have, by now, ironed out enough of the problems so that the program meets the needs of a reasonable cross section of patients.

I would like to apologize for the frequent use of the pronoun "he" in referring to diabetics when, in my limited experience, there seem to be more diabetic women than men. This is an unfortunate convention that has evolved in our language and is difficult to avoid without being inconsistent or cumbersome.

If you are reading this manual with the serious intention of using it as a guide for the treatment of insulin-dependent diabetes, *please read the footnotes*. Their location at the bottom of a page is usually a matter of editorial convenience and may be unrelated to the importance of their content.

Thank you.

Richard K. Bernstein
January 1981

1

THE UNNECESSARY TRAGEDY OF DIABETES

Most publications written for patients and their families paint a picture of diabetes as a mild inconvenience with certain long-term problems that can, usually, be avoided by the moderately conscientious patient. Articles by researchers and clinicians in the field, directed to their own colleagues, usually paint a far more grave and more accurate picture of the effects of this disease on the patient population.

According to recent data, diabetes is the third leading cause of death by disease in the United States—outranked by only cardiovascular ailments and cancer. Life span from the time of onset of diabetes is reduced by 30 percent for the average patient. The life span of insulin-dependent, or juvenile onset, diabetics, is reduced considerably more. Diabetes is the leading cause of new cases of blindness in the U.S. and a major cause of kidney disease, neurological disorders, cardiovascular morbidity, impotence, and nonaccidental amputation of limbs, to mention only a few of the major complications. The psychological damage that this disease has brought to patients and their families is of a magnitude beyond measure.

A recent study of 500 unselected diabetics, 92 percent of whom were insulin dependent, with an average disease duration of 9 years and a mean age of 29 years, showed 40 percent

1

with retinopathy, 52 percent with neuropathy, 13 percent with cataracts, 39 percent with kidney disease, 5 percent with coronary artery disease, 9 percent with peripheral vascular disease, and 34 percent with elevated blood lipids.[1]

The following typical story is especially sad in the light of our new-found knowledge that much of the suffering described can now be avoided.

Diabetes: A Personal Approach [2]
by Ellen Gerson [3]

I am 34 years old and have been diabetic since I was 11. I am also totally blind, having lost my sight as a direct result of diabetic retinopathy. I am continually learning to live with these problems, but in my gut I hate being blind and I hate being a diabetic.

Sometimes I think that if I had my choice (really not possible!), I would rather be blind than diabetic. With blindness, I more or less know what to expect. If I do not want to sit home and become a vegetable, I must get accustomed to the idea that although my eyes do not function, *I* must function. I must get out and live as active and as full a life as possible. I must make accommodations for my blindness, but I must live my life. I must face the frustrations of my blindness; things take longer for me to accomplish, are more devilish or inconvenient. But this is the way things are and I must get accustomed to it whether I like it or not.

But with diabetes, I must face the possibility of other complications—circulatory problems, infection and amputation, cardiovascular problems, kidney failure. And these complications may just happen, no matter how well I take care of myself. The way I perceive it is that with blindness, I more or less know what problems I need to face and I try to work them out as best I can. Diabetes, though, is a Sword of Damocles, and the unknown problems are doubly frightening *because* of their unknownness.

---

1. J. Achtenberg and A. Drexler. Experience with a Diabetic Registery, *Diabetes* 29: 130A (1980).

2. Courtesy *Journal of Visual Impairment and Blindness*, November 1978.

3. Ellen Gerson is a librarian, New York Public Library, Library for the Blind and Physically Handicapped.

I remember almost as if it were yesterday the events that took place when my family and I discovered I had diabetes. My mother, herself a diabetic, became concerned when I began to show some symptoms of diabetes and took me to our family doctor. When we returned a few days later to get the results of the tests, the doctor took my parents into his office while I waited outside. Finally I was asked to come in. I saw my mother with tears in her eyes, clutching a wet tissue in her hand. My father was not crying but had a rigid, frightened look on his face. I knew there was something terrible going on. When they told me that I had diabetes, I do not think I fully realized what it meant. But I knew it was "bad." Then the doctor told us that I would have to enter the hospital for "observation," which included more tests, regulation of my diet and insulin, and learning how to give myself insulin.

One of the more rotten things about my entering the hospital, aside from any child's fears about the hospital, was that I missed playing the lead role in my Hebrew School play—strike one against diabetes! But something else happened at the time of my hospitalization that had a great impact on me. I can only guess at the explanation for the events that followed.

My parents, or perhaps just my mother, never told any of my friends the real reason for my hospitalization. As far as any of them knew, I was in the hospital to have my appendix removed. Although I did not realize it then, the seeds of the idea that being a diabetic was something to be hidden were sown. I guess I began to be ashamed of myself.

Out of the Closet

My mother made other comments to me as I was growing up to indicate that I should not tell people that I was diabetic. I am sure that she thought she was doing what was best for me, that she was doing the right thing. Possibly her feelings grew out of her own experiences and what she had been told as she was growing up. Unfortunately, I carried these feelings with me into my early twenties when finally, after a serious illness when I could no longer hide my diabetes, I "came out of the closet."

Before this time, I had never told my friends, current or prospective employers, or colleagues that I was diabetic. But now I was admitting it—and stressful things were happening. I was prevented from obtaining a permanent New York City teacher's license because of my medical condition. Once I was refused summer employment at a large department store because I was diabetic. I was marked "different." At work, I was not able to donate blood. Who wanted a diabetic's blood? It was "bad" blood.

Each rebuff in my adult life served to reinforce my childhood memories and perceptions of what it was to be a diabetic. No one had ever been able to explain to me why I was not allowed to eat the goodies that my friends stuffed themselves with. Even now I love to eat, and it seems so unfair that, through no fault of my own, I should not eat the really delicious foods from all over the world.

When I was younger it seemed like such an effort to go away to visit friends, to go to camp, to go on vacation. I always had to make sure I had my medications and syringes. I had to make sure there were adequate medical facilities available. I had to make sure that the proper foods were available.

Even now, as I write this, I am enveloped in feelings of anger and frustration at the unfairness of the whole situation. Although my feelings about diabetes have mellowed as I mature, I still think that diabetes is a lousy disease. I have lost some close friends because of complications of diabetes. I know more and more people who have gone blind as a direct result of diabetes. I have many friends who have severe medical problems from diabetes-linked complications.

I used to think, and perhaps a part of me still does or would like to think, that diabetics can lead relatively normal lives if they take care of themselves. Unfortunately, I am not that optimistic any more. I feel strongly that the medical profession knows very little about diabetes and cannot predict what will or will not happen to a diabetic. But then, life itself is not very predictable.

If we use the tools and techniques now available to the diabetic, we can truly change the diabetic condition from a tragedy to an inconvenience. Ellen Gerson's story need no longer be repeated millions of times over. Chapter 4 contains comments by several diabetics who are no longer living under Ellen's "Sword of Damocles." The way out, however, requires serious initial commitment by the clinician and the patient.

2

WHY NORMALIZE BLOOD GLUCOSE?

by Samuel M. Rosen, M.D.

Clinical Director, Diabetes Research and Training Center of the Albert Einstein College of Medicine and Montefiore Hospital & Medical Center

When Dick Bernstein asked me to write an introductory chapter to this book, I was first tempted to develop a very scholarly document which would offer an argument supporting the value of tight control of blood sugar. It rapidly became apparent that his book was hardly the vehicle for an exhaustive review of the literature of the past forty years.

I have chosen to give a more personal view which has evolved from my roles as coordinator of undergraduate teaching in diabetes, as an internist with a small private practice devoted almost exclusively to diabetes, and as clinical director of a diabetes research and training center. In this last role, I have had the opportunity to plan education programs in diabetes for large numbers of internists and family physicians practicing sophisticated medicine in a major urban area.

During my fourth year of medical school, I attended a series of superb lectures by Dr. Robert Loeb, undoubtedly one of the great teachers in modern medicine. Dr. Loeb, at the time, pointed out that there were two conflicting schools of thought on diabetes care. The first held that control of blood sugar was of great importance in preventing the long-term complications of diabetes. The second believed that

5

these long-term consequences were independent of blood-sugar control. Dr. Loeb pointed out, quite correctly, that the data available at that time to support either position were quite thin and that one could not reach any justifiable conclusions. It is no wonder that my teachers chose to spend most of their time on the acute problems of the diabetic (for example, ketoacidosis), which are more easily treated, as well as studied.

During my internship and residency, my colleagues and I took comfort in an observation which was then (and, alas, still is) the conventional wisdom. We felt that it was not really important to resolve the question of blood-sugar control because most diabetics are in no way motivated to perform heroic maneuvers such as achieving ideal weight and taking 3–5 injections of Regular insulin each day. We all heard about small numbers of well-motivated diabetic physicians who were able to live with their disease for 20–40 years with little or no evidence of complications, but we were quick to realize that they comprised a small and highly select segment of the diabetic population. It is no wonder that my generation of physicians, and the generation that preceded us, developed a sense of futility about blood-sugar control that determined our medical practices for many years, which in turn affected the attitudes that we transferred to both our patients and our students.

Illustrative of the bewildering presentation of the tight control controversy are a pair of articles published in the prestigious *New England Journal of Medicine* four years ago. The first, a statement representing the official posture of the American Diabetes Association, reviewed a number of important studies which, on balance, provided important supportive evidence for the proponents of tight control. A few months later, a rebuttal to this position was written by a group of distinguished diabetologists who emphasized the inconclusive nature of many of the critical studies and pointed out the supposed dangers (largely hypoglycemia) of attempting to achieve tight control in the insulin-dependent diabetic, with the technology then available.

In view of the public disagreement among the experts on diabetes, it is no wonder that nonspecialists have, for the most part, taken the path of least resistance, believing that tight control may not carry with it rewards which justify the time, expense, and presumed risks. Furthermore, some have even made a virtue out of loose control. The number of patients who panic when their urine glucoses are negative is ample testimony to the misdirected viewpoint that derives, not from poor motivation in the patient, but from the mixed messages received from providers of health services. Another point of view that has pervaded medical practice is the belief that attempts at tight control, in an almost obligatory fashion, carry with them the probability of impaired psychological adjustment.

To my great satisfaction, a large group of diabetics are now prepared to take charge of their disease and are turning to physicians and other health advisors for guidance. There are, unfortunately, very few resources of real value to assist them in their task. I consider the present book a major addition to this category.

The balance of this chapter reviews some of the studies supporting tight control and concludes with the suggestion that the present state of our knowledge, plus recently developed technology, makes tight control both possible and safe for the average insulin-dependent diabetic.

The complications of diabetes that I will discuss are mainly those which are considered microangiopathic in origin—that is, they result primarily from thickening of the walls of the very small blood vessels throughout the body and culminate most importantly in severe involvement of the kidneys and the eyes. (Although the origin of the degeneration of peripheral nerves in diabetics may not be related to microvascular disease, many of the studies I cite also enable one to draw important inferences about the relationship of blood sugar to diabetic neuropathy.)

The exact correlation between glycemic (blood-sugar) control and another group of lesions which occurs with great frequency in diabetics is less clear. This group includes coronary artery disease, cerebral-vascular disease, and disease of the large blood vessels in the lower extremities. Although there is considerable evidence relating accelerated atherosclerosis (hardening of the arteries, the pathological lesion common to these diseases) to abnormal levels of certain fatty substances in the blood of poorly controlled diabetics, the precise nature of the origin of these lesions has not been elucidated.

From an important set of epidemiological studies it has become apparent that diabetics whose blood sugars are kept below 200 milligrams per deciliter (mg/dl) have significantly less diabetic retinopathy than do those with blood sugars above 200, but the former remained at risk to the ravages of coronary artery disease. One would like to know if the better-controlled group would also have been protected from atherosclerosis if their blood sugars were kept strictly within the normal range. Unfortunately, the answer to this question is not yet available.

Origin of Microangiopathic Lesions

Only a few reputable scientists continue to believe that the lesions of the small blood vessels (microangiopathy) are an inherent part of diabetes mellitus unrelated to the severity of the hormonal and metabolic alterations that characterize the diabetic state. This small group of scientists believes that abnormalities of small vessels are an intrinsic part of the process that produces diabetes and that changes in the basement membrane that supports these tiny vessels can precede the development of elevated blood sugars. It is only reasonable that the scientists espousing this point of view also believe that regulation of blood sugar would have no significant impact on the course of microangiopathy. This point of view, although not discredited entirely, continues to lose favor. Important evidence undermining this position comes from at least two sources. Identical twins by definition have a common genetic background. If diabetes develops in one member of a twin pair, the other has at least a 50 percent chance of developing diabetes. The unaffected twin does not appear to be at risk for the development of microvascular lesion unless he develops diabetes. This clearly indicates that the complications are somehow directly related to the diabetic state *per se* and not to any mysterious genetic factor independent of the diabetes.

Evidence against any mysterious factors unrelated to blood sugar is further supported in observation of diabetics receiving kidney transplants. In many of these cases, the transplanted kidneys coming from nondiabetic donors develop pathological lesions identical to those found occurring spontaneously in the diabetic. In these cases, it appears that elevated blood sugars (or other aspects of the abnormal chemical environment of the diabetic) are major, if not the only, determinants of diabetic complications.

Over the past ten years, a large number of careful studies have led to the conclusion that thickening of capillary blood vessel basement membranes, the anatomical basis of microangiopathy, is a function of the duration of diabetes and of the degree of control and not a phenomenon independent of altered glucose metabolism.

The thickened basement membrane is believed by most authorities to be a result of the binding of glucose (sugar) and its metabolic byproducts to the proteins that make up basement membrane. The simplest model that illustrates this process is reflected in a relatively new laboratory test—measurement of hemoglobin A_1C. Here, elevated glucose in the blood leads to the incorporation of part of the glucose molecule into the hemoglobin (a protein) of red blood cells. Although no major adverse effect of the change in composition of the hemoglobin molecule has been established, there appears to be some change in the ability of the hemoglobin to release oxygen. Accumulation of glucose derivatives into other important protein substances in the blood and other tissues has also been reported.

That accumulation of sugar can have serious effects is probably best illustrated in the eye. Here, glucose enters the lens and is converted to a substance called sorbitol. Since sorbitol cannot readily diffuse out of the lens, it accumulates and attracts water. The increase in the water content then leads to a disruption of the lens fibers and the formation of an opacity of the lens known as a cataract. Diabetics who are out of control seem to be prone to at least one specific form of cataract and in this case we can attribute a rather common complication of diabetes to blood-sugar elevation.

Let us briefly examine some of the evidence that control of blood sugar can either prevent or minimize the classical microangiopathic complications of diabetes.

Perhaps the most important studies in experimental animals are those of Bloodworth and his colleagues at the University of Wisconsin. Dogs were made diabetic by injections of a chemical which destroys the insulin-producing islets of Langerhans in the pancreas. Some of these newly diabetic dogs were subjected to a regimen which resulted in "good" control, while others were given enough insulin to survive, but with "poor" control. When the eyes, kidneys, and muscles of these animals were examined over a five-year period, the "good" control group had a dramatically lower rate of diabetic complications. In the case of eye lesions, the "good" control group was not much worse off than a group of nondiabetic animals. The purist can often find reasons to deny the relationship of the types of lesions found in the dogs to those of humans, but the comparability of the lesions, and the implications for therapy, seem to me most impressive.

It is important to note that the dogs used in these studies were not genetically destined to develop spontaneous diabetes, and that as far as we know, islet cell destruction, insulin deficiency, and hyperglycemia (high blood sugar) were the major factors distinguishing the diabetic animals from the controls. The differences detected in the incidence and severity of complications seen in the well-controlled group of animals versus those in the poorly controlled group imply, and (as far as I am concerned) prove, a cause-effect relationship between glycemic control and complications in the dog.

Mauer and his colleagues at the University of Minnesota have performed another series of simple yet elegant studies which establish that it is the elevated blood sugar and resultant abnormal levels of some important hormones that lead to the development of the lesions of diabetes in experimental rats. Kidneys from normal rats transplanted into diabetic animals developed lesions usually associated with diabetes in that species. Conversely, kidneys from diabetic animals transplanted into normals show a significant reversal of diabetic lesions. Once again, these clear-cut results provide strong evidence against the existence of mysterious tissue factors or genetically determined capillary thickening, independent of the blood glucose of the diabetic animal.

Population Studies in Humans

One would hope that data from studies of humans would provide evidence of the efficacy of glycemic control as convincing as that found in experimental animals. However, such definitive evidence is not yet available, and no large-scale well-controlled randomized clinical trial has yet been

performed. Accordingly, the only data derive from population studies (results of which can never unequivocally
demonstrate cause-and-effect relationships) and from retrospective studies of groups of patients, in which observer bias
and the presence of unknown nonrandomized risk factors
can significantly affect the results. No study has analyzed
results in any large group of patients who have been subjected to the degree of euglycemia (normal blood sugar level)
achievable with the tight control regimens that are now
being applied—using home glucose monitoring coupled with
either multiple-dose insulin regimens or with constant insulin infusion. However, even within the constraints of nonrandomized studies there is now a growing consensus that
the complications of diabetes are correlated with the duration and degree of impaired glycemic control.

The degree of control seems to be related not only to the
incidence of complications within a group of patients, but
also to the severity and rate of progression of these complications. In a prodigious study of 4,400 patients whom he personally followed over a 25-year period, the Belgian physician
Jean Pirart clearly demonstrated the relationship between
poor control and diabetic retinopathy, neuropathy, and
nephropathy (kidney disease).

A number of observers have commented on the relationship between the degree of control during the early years of
diabetes and the ultimate appearance of complications. This
has suggested that some significant changes may take place
in early diabetes that may markedly affect the later man-
ifestations of the disease.

On the other hand, the studies of Pirart and Johnsson suggest that, despite a long history of adequate control, a lapse
in control late in the course of the disease can precipitate
complications. These two positions are not incompatible.
There is no question that early in the course of diabetes there

are significant functional as well as structural changes in many of those tissues that may ultimately show classical diabetic lesions. In the course of early diabetes, for example, the kidney size is increased, and there are significant alterations in kidney blood-flow patterns years or decades before the kidney shows signs of clinical dysfunction. Microaneurysms, a characteristic lesion of diabetic retinopathy, can be detected by angiography within two or three years after the onset of childhood diabetes. Stephen Factor, of our institution, has recently been able to show the appearance of microaneurysms in the hearts of rats within six weeks after the induction of diabetes. Thus, it would appear that control of blood sugar during the early years of diabetes, as well as during critical periods, such as pubescence, can affect the ultimate outcome of the disease.

Effects of Tight Control in Early Diabetic Lesions

For a number of years it has been appreciated that certain functional abnormalities are present in early diabetes and are reversed with good control. Typical of this is increase in kidney size and evidence of abnormally high kidney filtration rates. In recent years, we have come to appreciate that other more subtle abnormalities are present and that these too can be completely or at least partially reversed by control of blood sugar.

In a recent preliminary study with which Dr. Bernstein was affiliated, a group of diabetics on a regimen similar to the one described in this book were tested for leakage of protein into the vitreous humor of the eye, using a highly sensitive new technique. This study provided important evidence suggesting that a three-month period of tight control resulted in a significant diminution of leakage. In another study examining the amount of protein excreted by the kidney, it was demonstrated that regulation of blood sugar is associated with a significant decline in the leakage of proteins from abnormal vascular beds. While the precise nature of the interrelationships of abnormal vascular permeability in the eye and kidney and the processes that culminate in significant compromise of ophthalmic and kidney function have not been firmly established, common sense leads me to believe that protein in the urine and protein leakage from the retina are reflections of the basic lesions of diabetic microangiopathy. Furthermore, it makes infinite sense to assume that maneuvers that can reverse these very subtle lesions could be beneficial in delaying, preventing, or in some cases reversing the development of the full-blown clinical complications.

It would be foolish to state that the efficacy of control in preventing or minimizing complications in humans has been absolutely proven. I believe that the body of evidence supporting tight control is now so convincing and the relationship between control and complications so fundamentally logical that the burden of proof rests squarely in the hands of the doubters. Although rats, dogs, and other experimental animals are not people, it is very difficult to conceive that the many well-controlled studies in these species are irrelevant to diabetes in humans.

It cannot be said that every diabetic who does not achieve ideal control is destined to develop complications. A significant number of diabetics are able to live with their disease for many decades without paying much or any attention to their degree of glycemic control and yet suffer few documented consequences of the diabetic state. A number of variables other than degree of control can affect the development of complications in a given patient. Genetic factors, plus risk factors such as hypertension and high levels of certain serum lipids, are likely to modify the effects of elevated blood sugar upon individual diabetics.

Until recently, even those of us who have accepted the

desirability of achieving tight control have been loath to recommend it to large numbers of our patients. Our concern about the supposed risks of hypoglycemia, our underlying prejudice that diabetics could not be motivated to take on the burden of multiple daily injections and major modifications in life style, paralyzed us for decades. More recently, we came to appreciate that most of those diabetics who we thought to be well controlled on conventional regimens, in reality have major fluctuations in blood sugar if several determinations are made over the course of the day. This frustration enhanced our belief in the futility of attempting to achieve a fine degree of control.

Dick Bernstein first came into my office two years ago. He told me about his recent admission to our medical school and asked if he could spend some of his spare time in our Diabetes Center. At first I was surprised that our admissions committee had accepted a 45-year-old "student." I assumed that he was another "professional" diabetic who thought he knew more than his doctors. However, I became intrigued by this brilliant and successful management engineer. He demonstrated how he had adapted to battery operation an electronic device for measuring blood sugar in the clinical laboratory, which we had previously regarded as useless. He had converted it to a portable instrument for home monitoring of blood glucose, long before reports in the British literature made self-monitoring fashionable. I was further taken aback to learn from associates that he had been teaching his method to distinguished physicians at other institutions, who, with his help, were successfully treating their more difficult patients.

To my eventual delight, I have established an extremely productive relationship with him. In this case, the clinician became the student and I began to learn his method, first from an early manuscript of this book and then with a group of my insulin-requiring patients who would meet with Dick and me every Sunday morning at his house. This proved to be one of the most stimulating educational experiences of my life.

I was initially very skeptical about a number of factors:

1. How could people prick their fingers 5–6 times a day?
2. Can one really expect a diabetic to take at least three injections of insulin a day, plus supplementary doses if blood sugar is elevated?
3. Could diabetics conform to a low-carbohydrate diet with all of its attendant restrictions?
4. How frequently would severe hypoglycemic reactions occur?

The answers became apparent to me within six months.

1. Finger sticks never once surfaced as a significant problem.
2. Multiple insulin injections were easily achieved.
3. The low-carbohydrate diet was difficult—but a number of attractive menus were available.
4. While a few minor hypoglycemic episodes were reported, none of the patients had any of the frequent and more severe incidents that they often had experienced on their previous regimens. The minor episodes of hypoglycemia that occurred were easily corrected without blood sugar overshoot by the candies that the patients carried. Moreover, the patients rapidly learned that many of the symptoms which they formerly attributed to hypoglycemia were neither true hypoglycemia nor did they represent major changes in blood sugar.

The method developed by Bernstein has a number of highly desirable features. If correctly applied, it gives the patient (and his physician) a thorough understanding of important mechanisms of his physiology: the effective time span of his regular insulin, the recognition of precisely how much a unit of regular insulin will lower his blood sugar, the intimate understanding of his ability to handle different kinds of food, the specific way in which exercise will lower (and in some cases raise) the blood sugar, and so on. This knowledge, when finally sorted out, makes a dramatic impact on the ability of the patient to regulate for himself the triad of insulin, diet, and exercise. Moreover, of the several methods in our experience that attempt tight control with home monitoring, Bernstein's method has proven to be the procedure best suited for achieving euglycemia.

At first, I was somewhat concerned about the sense of independence which, over a 3–4 month period, developed in my patients. I soon became adjusted to my new role. No longer was I the healer to these patients—I was their teacher and their guidance counselor. I suspect that many physicians will be somewhat threatened by the new role. They will take little comfort in the fact that the word "doctor" comes from the Latin for "teacher"—a fact usually communicated as part of the concatenation of platitudes at medical school commencement exercises. This new posture is undoubtedly necessary in caring for the patient with any chronic disease. It is especially necessary in diabetics, who require frequent modifications of regimen, in response to changes both in the external environment as well as in the patient's internal milieu.

There are still many unanswered questions. We still do not know what the goals of therapy should be. Is a blood sugar of 110 much better than one of 145? How widely applicable is this method? Can the nonspecialist become adept at it? Will very young children be able to adhere to the regimen? What kind of deviations from the method are tolerable?

The detailed description of the method in this manual will prove an invaluable guide to patients and physicians who are willing to devote the considerable amount of time and effort needed to achieve "physiologic" control. There is also little question that knowledge of the pathophysiology of diabetes, and of the individual responses to the disease and its therapy which will be achieved by following this manual, can serve as a useful springboard for further modification of the regimen by creative physicians and patients. This is entirely appropriate.

We are at the beginning of a new era in the management of diabetes in which many new approaches and technologies will be introduced. Bernstein's book offers, to motivated patients and health-care providers, what I believe to be the first really useful "how-to" introduction to the new technology.

While mastery of the GLUCOGRAF regimen initially requires many long hours on the parts of the patient and his health-care provider, the rewards of glycemic control and the anticipated prevention of grave sequelae justify the required effort.

3

AN OVERVIEW OF THE ENTIRE REGIMEN

SUMMARY

1. Major elements of the GLUCOGRAF regimen include:
   a. Patient performs at least six 1-minute blood glucose (BG) measurements daily.
   b. At least three small daily insulin doses before meals.
   c. Use of both long-acting and short-acting insulins.
   d. Correction of deviations from normal BG, made promptly and precisely—when high, by a precalibrated mini-dose of Regular insulin; when low, by one or more precalibrated sweets.
   e. A high-protein, very-low-carbohydrate diet, with total elimination of simple sugars except when exercising or for treatment of hypoglycemia.
   f. Measurement of glycosylated hemoglobin at least every few months.
2. Patient compliance with this regimen has been excellent.

Subsequent chapters detail and explain the various facets of the GLUCOGRAF regimen. There is some value in first summarizing the entire approach, with very little clarification or explanation. This will enable the reader later to fit each step, as it arises, into the overall framework of treatment set forth in this chapter. It may also relieve some curiosity and perhaps enlighten those who were hoping that the goal of normal blood sugars could be attained without dedication and effort.

Our system was worked out by trial and error and will require some experimentation for every patient. Its basic goal is to maintain normal blood glucose (BG) levels throughout every day and night. The technique attempts to have the patient mimic as closely as possible both the insulin activity of the normal pancreas and the counter-regulation (prevention of very low BG levels) that occurs in nondiabetics. This is to be accomplished with total daily insulin doses that, in most cases, will not exceed what is produced naturally by the nondiabetic pancreas.

The basic regimen, for most patients, contains the following 7 elements:

1. At least three small daily doses of insulin—one dose prior to every meal. The morning and evening doses will probably be mixtures of long-acting insulin (usually Ultralente) and rapid-acting insulin (usually Regular). The midday dose will usually entail just Regular insulin. The injections will be given far enough in advance of each meal so that the Regular insulin begins to enter the bloodstream at the same time that glucose produced by digestion of foodstuffs also begins to enter the bloodstream.

2. Simple sugars, such as those contained in many desserts, candies, and fruits, will be totally eliminated from the diet, except for treatment of hypoglycemia (low BG levels) and during periods of exercise. Most dietary carbohydrate will be replaced by protein, which is converted to BG much less rapidly. In most patients, carbohydrate will be limited to

no more than one bread exchange [1] per meal. There will be no snacks between meals, except under special conditions to be described. It will, however, be possible to eliminate or reschedule any meals, provided that the appropriate dose of Regular insulin is similarly eliminated or rescheduled.

3. The patient will not test urines for sugar but will, instead, measure his BG directly at least 6 times per day. The BG test requires a simple finger prick and one drop of blood. The simple equipment for measuring BG is described in Chapter 8. The test takes only 1 or 2 minutes to perform and requires no special technical capability.

4. The patient will learn how to calibrate the amount that 1 unit of insulin will lower his BG. Whenever his BG test is even slightly elevated, he will immediately take exactly the right amount of Regular insulin to bring the BG down exactly to an ideal level (usually 100 mg/dl).

5. Whenever a patient feels the earliest symptoms of a possible low BG, he will immediately perform a one minute BG test. If his BG is lower than the ideal level, he will take exactly the right number of glucose tablets or small candies to bring his BG back up to exactly the ideal point, without "overshoot."

6. The patient will learn how to prevent hypoglycemia, during or after exercise, without causing excessive elevation of BG. This will involve some BG measurements before and after a typical exercise session and the simple computation of how often a standard glucose tablet or candy must be eaten while exercising.

7. Follow-up laboratory determinations of glycosylated hemoglobin levels (see Chapter 7) should be conducted at least every few months so that the physician can check the success of the patient's efforts.

---

1. "Bread exchange" is the basic unit of measure for complex carbohydrates. See Chapter 13 (footnote page 156) and Appendix A.

It should be obvious from the preceding that our regimen is considerably more complex than the simple set of rules usually taught to newly diagnosed insulin-dependent diabetics. Therefore it would be unwise for the average patient to begin without *close professional supervision*. This means telephone calls from the patient to the physician (or other health care professional) at least once daily, during the first two weeks of the new treatment. The initial burden on the physician is more than compensated for by the eventual independence [2] that the patient gains, after he has perfected his skills of self-regulation.

Most patients adjust best to the new regimen if, after 1–2 weeks of practice in measuring their own BG, they are switched over to all 7 of the previously described elements *simultaneously*. The new insulin regimen, for example, will not lead to reasonable BG values, unless the dietary changes are incorporated at the same time. Gradual changes in regimen will delay the onset of continuously normal BG. This delay is very frustrating to a patient who is measuring BG and knows that it is fluctuating over an abnormal range. He wants results and the sooner he gets them, the more likely he will be to comply with the regimen.

Some physicians, upon seeing this list of 7 elements, have said, "I can't ask a patient to take three daily injections and six daily finger pricks." Any number of patients have already replied, "Let us decide for ourselves; we're the ones who are facing early death and disability. Maybe it's worth a try." For further comments relating to patient compliance see Appendix C of this manual (Dr. Robert Tattersall's editorial from *Diabetologia*) and the firsthand experiences described in Chapter 4.

---

2. This new independence need not cause the physician to lose patients. Indeed, the handful of physicians using this method are actually retaining grateful patients and attracting new ones by virtue of their reputations for being able to control an "uncontrollable" disease.

4

BEFORE AND AFTER—
FIVE PATIENTS RECALL THEIR FEELINGS

Five people, now controlling their insulin-dependent diabetes according to their own variations of the method described in this manual, were asked to answer two questions:

1. What were your principal feelings and day-to-day thoughts about your diabetes before you were able to normalize your blood glucose levels?

2. What are your current feelings, including those relating to taking several daily injections, pricking your finger, restricting your diet, and being obliged continually to recognize the effects of your activities upon blood sugar?

These people come from a variety of socioeconomic and educational backgrounds, have been diabetic for differing lengths of time, and have varying degrees of diabetic complications (including none). Their comments are self-explanatory. It is interesting to note how their personal revelations present certain common themes.

Ellen B. Lanners

"I became a person again. I am now in control of my life."

Mrs. Lanners is a 40-year-old electron microscopist known to have been diabetic for the past 19 years. She produces endogenous insulin, and is now injecting only 5 units daily, divided among 3 pre-meal doses. She has been on the regimen for 3 years.

Before I embarked upon this program I felt totally overwhelmed by both physical and emotional problems which seemed to affect every aspect of my existence. I felt "sick" most of every day, except when doing something very physically demanding, like pulling a loaded shopping cart or hiking in the mountains for eight hours, which, I guess, brought down my blood sugar.

Emotionally I was plagued by my constant inability to concentrate or formulate ideas. I was often confused and impatient, as well as aggressive and even hostile to those around me. Since I was unable to establish any personal goals, I completely lost my feeling of self-worth.

None of this was helped by my poor relationship with my diabetologist. Although the doctor was patient, listened carefully, and encouraged me to call him at home if I needed to, I always left his office feeling frustrated and anxious, because we really weren't getting anywhere. My complaints of always feeling ill had little credibility. The only documentation I had was 2+ and 3+ urine test results, and the feeling of hypoglycemia perhaps twice in any 24-hour period. These facts, combined with the results of the doctor's tests, did not give us sufficient information to suggest changes in either the timing or dosage of insulin. Although the idea of accurately determining my own blood glucose levels over a 24-hour period had occurred to me, I didn't know that this was actually possible, and I felt continually miserable because I couldn't straighten out my life. Even worse, I felt totally dependent on the doctor despite the fact that he didn't seem able to help me.

These burdens occupied 90 percent of my waking hours. As a result, my relationship with my husband, as well as with others, suffered. My husband couldn't understand why I felt so helpless and hopeless, and most of my family and friends thought my problem was an emotional one, having to do with a lack of goals and difficulty with authority figures. As a result of this lack of understanding, I was left with great feelings of inferiority and even felt that people were hostile toward me.

From the moment I started with this new approach, I felt challenged and gratified that I could finally exercise some definitive measures that had positive results. I found that I was easily able to fit the details of the new regimen into my life. Now I perform these tasks almost automatically, without even thinking about them. I was never bothered by pricking my finger, and divided small doses of insulin are certainly less painful to inject than a single big dose. Adjusting the insulin amount and the proper timing has worked out perfectly 90 percent of the time, and while I can't always find a private room in which to do it, a sense of humor and determination always see me through. Actually I was once disappointed to find that no one seemed to notice as I measured out and injected my insulin in a busy public laundromat. Certainly motivation has a lot to do with it, and the rewards have been immense.   4, 4 - 5. 6

I am now able to maintain a blood glucose level of 80–100 mg/dl, and the longer I adhere to this regimen the more even nonroutine situations become a challenge which I know my experience can overcome. I no longer feel stressed or insecure with regard to my diabetes.

A second benefit has been my ability to document my condition in the doctor's office. With my brief daily notes on insulin amounts and timing, when and which foods consumed, exercise, stress, and illness, the doctor has a basis on which to ground his decisions. We are now co-workers in solving questions with respect to my health. I am in a better position to understand his suggestions. In fact, I am more familiar with my body's reactions than the doctor is. There have been times when I have modified his suggestions with great success. I am now in control of my life. This has brought back my self-esteem. Those who love and care about me now feel relieved. They support me most enthusiastically.

To summarize my feelings, no element of the program I follow presents a burden for me. The reason is very clear: Before, no aspect of my existence was positive. I could not accept the fact that there was no way out except that of not existing. Given the materials and methods to climb out of that condition, is it surprising that all those details became almost completely automatic for me? I became a person again. I am a winner in the most basic aspects of living and I've been freed to strive for the many challenges which life presents.

J.C.

"This regimen gives *you* the tools to take charge of *your* body."

J.C. became diabetic at age 13½. Prior to going on tight blood glucose control, he had developed osteoporosis, which eventually led to a fractured arm that did not heal properly. He had also developed diabetic retinopathy for which he received laser treatments. Further retinal deterioration does not seem to have occurred since he has been on the regimen. He is now 25, with a life-style markedly less disciplined and more frenetic than those of the other cases presented here.

Four years ago my diabetes was well under control *on paper.* My charts and records showed mostly normal urines but actually I was cheating quite a lot. I would then take extra insulin to bring down my elevated blood sugars before going to the doctor's office. My troubles really began when I tried to bring myself under control. Hypoglycemic reactions were becoming a daily occurrence at my fast-paced job as a short-order cook. My emotional state was so low that at one point I tried to take my life by injecting three bottles of Regular insulin. It was a short time after this episode that I fortunately was recruited by some other diabetics into a program of tight blood glucose control.

On this new regime, I discovered the importance of taking daily multiple blood sugars and multiple insulin injections, coupled with a radically new diet and strenuous exercise. As they say, "Nothing worthwhile comes easy." This is certainly true of the program. You must become aware of the countless things that affect your body. You must develop a sense of timing, using forethought, and maintaining discipline. It is not an easy regimen to master in the beginning. Several tear-filled days were spent before I was on the right track. But if you have the determination and drive, you will succeed.

This regimen gives you the tools to take charge of your body.

With the meter you always know what your blood sugar is, and the program teaches you how to correctly compensate for high and low readings with either insulin or sugar.

Some people say that this program takes too long to learn and that pain must necessarily be involved in sticking your finger or multiple injections; however, this is not true. For me the pain came long before, from not knowing what my body was doing or how to treat it correctly.

The time spent in learning this new technique is not as considerable as one would think. As I see it, it is your own body, so you might as well learn the right way to care for it. I am now able to live my crazed and fast-paced life while still having control of my blood sugars.

Deborah Sloan

"I was always so frustrated and angry because the doctors kept telling me I was fine."

Ms. Sloan is a 37-year-old office manager.

About 12 years ago, at the age of 25, I was told that I had diabetes. At first I said, "I'll do what I'm told and everything will be fine," and I stuck to my diet and did the urine testing and some exercise and I tried to deal with the fact that I had a chronic disease. I had negative urine sugar all the time and a pretty good fasting blood sugar, and the doctors told me that I should feel well. But as the disease progressed I had to admit to myself that I was not feeling at all well. I was constantly tired—really badly fatigued, and often worried that I would go into shock. Since I had no energy, I felt as if I had no reason to go on—actually I felt as if I was on my way out. I was always so frustrated and angry because the doctors kept telling me I was fine.

What I eventually found out was that my renal threshold [1] was very high. I could be negative in the urine while my blood sugar was really anywhere from 250 down to 40. I was always fighting this, and because I was trained to eat if there was any doubt, I was always eating and ending up with high sugars.

---

1. Blood sugar value at which glucose first appears in the urine.

One day when I was visiting a new doctor, he did a blood-glucose test and told me I was at 315 and that that accounted for my feeling so bad. After watching him prick my finger and do the test, I asked him why I couldn't do that myself, and he said, "You can." Quite frankly, at that point I would have gladly pricked my finger 16 times a day if it would have meant controlling my blood sugar. For anyone used to taking insulin injections, sticking your finger is nothing terrible. So I started in a program of tight blood-glucose control and at this point I've been on the meter almost two years, and the fatigue, frustration, and all the problems that went with it are gone. I'm able to maintain my blood sugar between 65 and 130 milligrams almost without exception. Since my insulin is broken down into several small doses, it's a very small shot and I use my entire abdomen, hips, thighs, and arms. I have no problem at all. I wouldn't give up the regimen for anything. And as far as the expense, when you consider that I've avoided the usual hospitalizations, prevented complications, and am prolonging my life, I'd say it's more than justified! I certainly wish that I had known about this at the onset of my symptoms. Now I feel like a whole human being again! My life is back to where it was before I became a diabetic.

Dr. Paul Shevin

"After I began the GLUCOGRAF regime—what a change!"

Dr. Paul Shevin is a 46-year-old podiatrist practicing in Rye, New York, who has had diabetes since he was 21. At the age of 37, he suffered a myocardial infarction.[2] For one year prior to his starting on our regimen he was suffering from very painful and continuous neuropathy of his feet. The pain has now subsided, leaving a residual paresthesia[3] which may take from one to two years to reverse—if it does reverse.

For twenty-five years I felt as if I were on a rudderless ship, allowing my body to deteriorate. I was experiencing complica-

2. Heart attack.
3. Strange feeling.

tions involving retinopathy and neuropathy but I persisted in my belief that near-normal blood sugar levels were unobtainable. I had also been conditioned to think that this lack of control allowed for a carefree life style in which you "forgot" about your diabetes, but because of my medical training, I don't think I ever fully accepted that theory.

After I began the new regimen—what a change! While there is no question that it does make you constantly aware of your condition, and it does take a minimal amount of time to monitor your blood sugar, after a while all the monitoring and calculating become almost automatic. After all, man is a highly adjustable animal. And it's the only method available at the present time that allows an insulin-dependent diabetic to come close to living a full and normal life.

Utilizing this regime, I was even able to develop a highly effective weight-loss crash diet for myself that brought quick results. After a few days, there was no constant hunger, a rapid weight loss, and close to normal glycemia. Before this, no diabetic with a need for 3 meals a day plus snacks could have imagined in his wildest dreams being on such a diet!

There is no question that the Bernstein regimen as a whole works. I'm truly better now—both mentally and physically. For the first time I feel in command of my life. I am captain of my own ship.

Clara Ducham

"For 18 years I had very little indication of when an insulin reaction would occur. My biggest fear was being alone."

Ms. Ducham is secretary to the comptroller of a major manufacturer of medical equipment. She is 29 years old and has been diabetic since the age of 7. Her 16-year-old brother, Ken, also has diabetes. Clara suffered from a transient period of diabetic neuropathy while in college, and prior to being introduced to our regimen had laser treatments for retinal hemorrhages in one eye. Fortunately, her retinopathy appears to have been arrested without significant loss of vision.

Clara now spends her spare time working for the New York Diabetes Association where she teaches other diabetics how to measure their blood sugars.

My biggest fear was being alone. Behind that lay a fear of not being able to take care of myself. An insulin reaction would multiply these feelings to incredible levels of intensity. For eighteen years, I had very little way of knowing when a reaction would occur. I tried simple measures like eating a piece of fruit before exercising, but there were many other situations in which I could not act quickly enough to fend off the debilitating feeling brought on by low blood sugar.

One incident, in particular, will vividly reveal some of the difficulties involved in dealing with diabetes. One night after work, I was joining some friends to go to a baseball game at Yankee Stadium. I stopped to take insulin and have dinner and proceeded to the stadium. The game that night was between the Yankees and my beloved Boston Red Sox. During the top of the seventh inning, I started to feel shaky, but attributed it to the excitement of the game. By the top of the eighth inning, there wasn't any doubt in my mind. I ate a piece of candy. I didn't feel it was helping, so I asked my friend if she had any candy. She gave me what she had, but something was very wrong. Nothing seemed to make me feel any better at all. At the end of the game, I told my friends they would have to wait to leave because I had lost all feeling in my legs and didn't think I could climb down all the stairs from our general admission seats. At that point, one of the stadium security guards ordered us to clear out. My friends explained the situation to him and tried to enlist his help, but he decided that I must be one of those kids who had had a beer too many and was trying to be obnoxious. The situation came to a head when I passed out. When I came around, I was exiting the stadium via a litter carried by four security guards. One of my friends was muttering to me that I had missed meeting Bobby Murcer.

I would have loved to meet Mr. Murcer, but that was the least of my worries. Aside from the obvious embarrassment, more important and immediate was the fact that I had lost consciousness and there had been a lapse of time before I received medical attention. I think it is fortunate that I do tell my friends about my medical status, rather than trying to hide a condition that has to become apparent to anyone who spends time with me. What is unfortunate is that most diabetics have had very similar experiences. What haunts me to this day is that I did lose consciousness and for a period of time, however brief, was not able to take care of myself.

However, I'm not the kind of person who will let my diabetic condition hinder me from doing the things that I want to do. All diabetics live with a host of fears ranging from a shortened life span to worries about the quality of life and anxieties about whether they will be able to produce children.

One of the biggest questions I faced over the years was whether I have a right to have a baby when there is such a strong possibility that the baby might be a diabetic or his or her descendants might inherit the trait. Until recently, my answer was that I did not have the right and it made me feel very inadequate as a woman as well as discouraged about the narrowing options of my life. However, after 3 years on this regimen during which my diabetes and my general health improved I changed my mind. I became convinced that even if my child were a diabetic, he or she would probably be healthy and well cared for because of what I have learned about diabetes and fitness. While I would certainly rather the child weren't diabetic, I feel he or she would learn to take care of the situation, and also learn to handle the other aspects of life. In fact, he or she would probably do as well as, if not better than, many other people, because of having both the knowledge and the incentive to care for his or her body. I feel strongly that anyone who learns to deal with the variables involved in diabetes has a fundamental structure for learning to handle many other situations.

Since I have been using this method of controlling blood glucose, I have been able to take stock of my physical condition, deal successfully with it, and improve my self-esteem and have also alleviated a considerable amount of fear. I think my attitudes toward insulin injections, diet, and exercise reflect this general ability to cope with the many difficult situations, which I have just discussed. I was diabetic for several years before I learned to take care of injecting myself.

When I was a young diabetic, neither my parents nor I knew about the importance of rotating injection sites. We always used my arms and I ended up with a severe case of atrophy. The doctor finally told us not to use the arms at all, but to use the legs for a time. My arms did get somewhat better, but I always felt ashamed of their appearance, and was further upset when I developed both atrophy and hypertrophy in my legs. I have since learned about and practiced rotation of injection sites. Now that I am on the new regimen, by taking *small* doses of insulin several times each day and exercising regularly, I have been able to achieve nearly 100 percent improvement in the atrophy.

There was also a change in my attitude toward injections. Before I started home blood-glucose monitoring, I took two injections daily, before breakfast and before dinner. Soon after starting to monitor, I began taking three injections, adding a dose before lunch. Once I got used to the idea, I was willing to admit that indeed, this routine of mimicking a normally functioning pancreas was working well for me. In fact, my overall daily dosage was less than before. Besides the obvious advantage of better control, there is the reassurance, for me, that even if I do have a reaction as a result of some unexpected development, there is a smaller amount of insulin to deal with at any one time. The risks and discomforts of a reaction are thus minimized. Any diabetic will be able to back me up when I say that this is very comforting at 3:00 A.M. when I've awakened because of a reaction. I can measure my blood sugar, correct it with a small amount of carbohydrate, and fall back to sleep within a half-hour, rather than lie awake tossing and turning for two or three hours.

Now I not only poke myself several times each day to inject insulin, but since I began home blood-glucose monitoring, I poke my fingertips six or eight times each day. It took considerable powers of persuasion on the part of my doctors, but I was intrigued with the opportunity of checking my own blood sugar at any time. I used to tell my doctors that I thought my blood sugar level ranged too much over the course of a day. After they took a single blood sugar in the office and found it was "within normal limits," they would pat me on the back and dismiss me, implying, if not directly stating, that I was too much of a worrywart. Now I don't have to worry that my tiredness may be the beginning of an insulin reaction nor do I have to wait until I get to the doctor's office to find out what my condition really is.

It took me some time to decide to go this route. First of all, it certainly is not a pleasant idea for anyone to have to stick oneself. Second, I was concerned about the amount of damage I'd do to the nerve endings in the fingertips. Again, I have to admit that, happily, there has been little, if any, problem. In fact, nerve conduction studies done on me have shown improvement since I started this program of home monitoring. After three years of "finger poking," my attitude is that I can live with a certain amount of mild discomfort because I'm gaining the benefits of health and satisfaction in being able to take good care of myself.

Parenthetically, I can cite an example of how monitoring has saved me a fair amount of hassle. I've known for years that my blood sugar has a tendency to drop during the afternoon. A number of times when I've been very busy at work and found myself feeling tired, I've had the sense to take those few minutes to check my blood sugar. By finding the level and correcting it on the spot, I've saved myself and my co-workers a lot of aggravation.

In the area of diet, too, I think I have learned to cope better than some people who are 20 pounds overweight. That's not to say that diet isn't a problem. What I am saying is that I have a different perspective on the subject. I think many diabetics, as well as their dieticians, would like to banish the words "diet" and "cheating" from the English vocabulary. I prefer the expression "meal plan"—that is, the combination of foods that makes me feel best. This term also implies that I am making very conscious choices of what I am putting into my body. Since I've begun the new program, I've been increasingly better able to determine exactly what combinations work best for me. It has also helped me to adjust my insulin dosage for those social occasions when I want to be "part of the crowd" and enjoy something outside of my ordinary meal plan. I should interject a few words here because I'm sure any number of people who are reading this will say, "So, what we come down to is that home glucose monitoring offers the perfect out for cheating." I'm the last person to advocate that. However, I haven't met a person yet who has never departed from his usual "diet" at some point. With the ability to monitor blood sugar levels closely, the diabetic can take over more of the role that his pancreas, if functioning normally, would have automatically performed for him. Accordingly, with this program, we can alleviate some of the feelings of guilt, stress, and frustration that adversely affect diabetic control.

In summary, I can certainly say that the disciplined overall approach of my program has greatly improved the quality of my life. Since diabetes not only affects millions of patients but their families, friends, and business associates as well, I feel that the ramifications of this method of blood glucose control are extremely significant.

Some physicians have said that they don't want their patients to be burdened by thoughts relating to the control of their diabetes because such thoughts are "unnatural," or "unhealthy," or just an "unnecessary burden." We have not encountered any studies of the amount of time that insulin-dependent diabetics, not on our regimen, spend thinking about the control of blood-glucose swings but we suspect that it is considerable. A recent tabulation of the time spent, by a small group of patients with partial loss of vision, discussing various subjects during group psychotherapy sessions, follows.

COMPARISON OF ISSUES DISCUSSED BY DIABETICS DURING GROUP THERAPY

Issues	Time Consumed (percent)	Issues	Time Consumed (percent)
1. DIABETIC CONTROL	11.34	6. Group issues	6.52
2. Diabetic complications/fear of death	10.22	7. Reaction of family and friends	6.30
3. Diabetic retinopathy/loss of vision	9.06	8. Depression	4.60
4. Mobility	8.74	9. Suicide	4.04
5. Glaucoma/enucleation of eye	8.69	10. Rehabilitation agencies	3.98
		11. Dating/marriage/children	3.62

Issues	Time Consumed (percent)	Issues	Time Consumed (percent)
12. Career	3.52	pendence conflict	1.33
13. Stigma and prejudice of public	3.48	19. Limbo (due to fluctuating vision)	1.17
14. Reading	3.24	20. Anger	1.10
15. Fear of total blindness	2.82	21. Guilt	0.88
16. Hope	2.30	22. Group leader	0.32
17. Recreation	1.75	23. Finances	0.30
18. Independence/de-		24. Low-vision clinics	0.28
		25. Hospitalization	0.22

Oehler-Giarratana, J., and Fitzgerald, R.G. Group Therapy with Blind Diabetics, *Archives of General Psychiatry* 37:463–467 (1980).

Thus, among these patients who, some might think, have a more pressing problem—that is, imminent blindness—the number one subject for discussion was DIABETIC CONTROL. See Chapter 18 if you find it difficult to understand why this is so often the case.

5

THE ROLES OF CERTAIN HORMONES IN REGULATING BLOOD GLUCOSE LEVEL

SUMMARY

To ensure the continuous availability of glucose to the brain, the body utilizes chemical messengers, called hormones, that are released into the bloodstream. Certain "counter-regulatory" hormones stimulate the conversion of a stored starch (glycogen) and of stored proteins into blood glucose (BG). Digestion of large meals causes the secretion of counter-regulatory hormones from cells in the intestines. Increased BG levels are opposed by insulin which enables glucose to leave the blood and to enter the cells of various tissues. If insulin is not present, BG will rise, even if an individual fasts or eats foods that cannot be broken down to glucose.

It is the purpose of this chapter to give the reader an understanding of the major physiologic mechanisms that in the nondiabetic regulate blood glucose levels (BG) and provide the cells of the body with fuel. Most of these mechanisms also operate in the diabetic but are thwarted by an absent or ineffective insulin response. By learning how the normal body functions, we can better comprehend the measures that must be taken to maintain a comparable degree of regulation in the diabetic, and will also have the background to differentiate between the various types of diabetes described in Chapter 6. This is important since the approach to treatment differs for each type of diabetes.

Many tissues in the body are capable of storing fuels which can eventually be converted to energy. When stored, these fuels can take the forms of fats, protein (as in muscle tissue) and a starchy substance called glycogen. Both protein and glycogen can, under the direction of certain hormones, be transformed (usually in the liver) to BG. BG, in turn, can be rapidly utilized for the production of energy. The mechanisms for retrieving glucose from glycogen and protein are respectively called glycogenolysis and gluconeogenesis. These processes are especially necessary for the maintenance of life because the brain usually relies for its minute-to-minute existence on the blood glucose content. Because a supply of glucose can be of critical importance to survival of the brain in emergencies, the body is provided with a number of means for stimulating glycogenolysis and gluconeogenesis. These means all involve the release of so-called counter-regulatory hormones. Many counter-regulatory hormones work constantly, stimulating the elevation of BG. They are opposed by only one hormone, insulin.

The Pancreatic Hormones

The human body can utilize several fuels to supply energy for its many functions. The major fuel used by most body cells, most of the time, is a sugar called glucose (also called dextrose). In order for glucose to enter a cell or to enter smaller compartments within cells, there must be present, bound to the outside wall or membrane of the cell or compartment, a hormone called insulin. In untreated diabetes, insulin may be either totally absent from the cell membrane, present in inadequate amounts, or inadequately bound to receptor sites on the membrane. In any of these cases, glucose cannot be utilized effectively.

Insulin is a protein, manufactured and stored in an abdominal organ called the pancreas. Most of the tissue in the pancreas produces digestive juices (enzymes) that are released through narrow ducts into the small intestine. The tissue producing these enzymes is called exocrine or acinar tissue. Scattered sparsely throughout the exocrine tissue are tiny bits of endocrine (as opposed to exocrine) tissue called islets of Langerhans. These islets or islands are about the size of pinheads and release hormones directly into the bloodstream—not into the intestines. Hormones are chemical messengers that regulate processes at various locations in the body, which may be quite distant from the source of the hormone. The islets are, in turn, composed of at least four different types of cells (A, B, D, and F)—each producing at least one hormone. All of these hormones may have effects upon blood glucose, as summarized in the following table.

Type of Islet Cell	Hormone Produced	Effect upon Blood Glucose
A-cell (also called alpha cell)	Glucagon	Raises BG.
B-cell (also called beta cell)	Insulin	Lowers BG.
D-cell (also called delta cell)	Somatostatin	Limits extreme BG fluctuations by shutting off A-cells and B-cells in response to high or low BG levels.
	Gastrin	Appears to work in opposition to somatostatin, by stimulating the secretions of A- and B-cells. In diabetes, with dis-

Type of Islet Cell	Hormone Produced	Effect upon Blood Glucose
		abled B-cells, gastrin would raise BG via the unopposed A-cells.
F-cell	Pancreatic polypeptide	May regulate certain digestive secretions in the stomach and in the exocrine cells of the pancreas. Blood levels of this hormone are reduced in obese individuals, suggesting that it may also regulate the affinity of insulin receptors.

In the B-cells, insulin is manufactured and stored in microscopic granules. In a nondiabetic, when BG is elevated (as after a meal), the B-cells release some or all of the stored insulin to the bloodstream. If BG remains somewhat elevated, the B-cells will manufacture new insulin and release it as soon as it is ready. The response of the B-cell is therefore called biphasic—that is, an immediate release of stored insulin (phase I), followed by a slower release of newly manufactured insulin, over an extended time period (phase II).

Insulin causes a lowering of BG in at least four ways:

1. It permits most body cells to absorb glucose from the blood, and may also be involved in the process by which cells extract energy from glucose (metabolism). Certain cells, however, such as brain cells, nerves,[1] the lens of the eye, and special kidney cells appear to utilize glucose without the help of insulin.

2. It enables the liver to store glucose in the form of glycogen—a starch consisting of many glucose molecules attached to one another. The manufacture of glycogen by the liver is called glycogenesis. Muscles can also manufacture and store glycogen, but only in very small amounts.

---

1. Recent evidence supports the possibility that insulin may also serve one or more functions in nerve cells and in special sites within the brain.

3. It facilitates the conversion of excess glucose to fat, for storage as a long-term energy reserve.

4. It inhibits the conversion of amino acids to glucose in the liver, by facilitating their assembly into body proteins. Amino acids appear in the blood as a result of digestion of dietary proteins, breakdown of exercised muscle tissue, and other processes.

In addition, insulin enables fat cells to manufacture body fat from the fatty acids that enter the bloodstream after digestion of dietary fats.

Insulin, in summary, is a hormone that causes or facilitates the building of tissue. The process of building tissue is called anabolic metabolism.

On the other hand, the hormone glucagon, produced by the A-cells, facilitates catabolic metabolism—the breakdown of tissue into its building blocks. It is called a counter-regulatory hormone because it functions counter to insulin and serves to oppose excessive lowering of BG. Specifically, glucagon signals the liver to break down its stored glycogen to the glucose building blocks and to break down proteins in the blood to their component amino acids. The liver, influenced by glucagon, will even convert amino acids to glucose. This process whereby proteins are converted to glucose is called gluconeogenesis. Glucagon, when produced excessively, also influences cellular breakdown of fats into fatty acids and glycerol (a process called lipolysis). Fatty acids can be used by the body as fuel, but their oxidation as fuel produces toxic substances called ketonic acids and ketones. (One of these ketones, acetone, is the principal ingredient of nail-polish remover.) Glucagon will not serve all of these counter-regulatory functions if an excess of insulin is present.

The secretion of glucagon by the A-cells influences the B-cells to produce more insulin. Insulin, in turn, signals the A-cell to produce less glucagon. All the while, the D-cells may be producing somatostatin, which slows the secretion of both insulin and glucagon, or gastrin, which stimulates secretion of the two hormones. In the nondiabetic, the three types of cells work harmoniously to maintain BG over a very narrow normal range—neither too low nor too high.

The Adrenal Hormones

Located on the upper surfaces of the two kidneys are a pair of small endocrine glands called the adrenals. Some of the hormones they produce can help raise BG and, like glucagon, are frequently released in response to low BG levels. The adrenal hormones of interest to us are of two general types: the glucocorticoids and the catecholamines.

The glucocorticoids are produced by the outer part of the adrenal, called the cortex. They have a chemical structure similar to that of cholesterol and have names such as cortisone, corticosterone, hydrocortisone, etc. They are produced in response to certain types of stress and enhance the breakdown of amino acids (from protein) to glucose (gluconeogenesis). They also stimulate formation of glucose by the breakdown of glycogen, stored in the liver and muscles (glycogenolysis). At least some of these catabolic effects are mediated by a reduction in insulin binding sites.

The catecholamines (adrenalin and noradrenalin) are produced by the central portion of the adrenal, called the medulla. These are the "fight or flight" hormones that activate the body in times of danger or extreme physical stress (like competitive running). They stimulate many functions, including heart rate and conversion of glycogen to glucose in muscles and liver. They also facilitate the aforementioned breakdown of free fatty acids and inhibit insulin release from the B-cell.

Hormones secreted by other endocrine glands—such as neurotensin and the growth hormones—may tend to raise BG but usually are less important than the pancreatic and adrenal hormones already discussed.

Enteric (Intestinal) Hormones

The stomach and the small intestine contain many endocrine cells that secrete a variety of hormones into the bloodstream as a meal is being digested. A number of these "enteric" hormones have indirect effects upon BG, and several of them are also secreted by other organs such as the pancreas and the pituitary gland. For example:

Enteric Hormone	Effect upon BG
Enteroglucagon	Probably raises BG via the same biochemical pathways (for example, glycogenolysis) that are stimulated by glucagon.
Secretin	Mimics glucagon.
Somatostatin	Suppresses both insulin and glucose secretion from the pancreas.
Gastrin	Stimulates pancreatic secretion of insulin (from normal B-cells) and glucagon.
Cholecystokinin	Affects BG similarly to gastrin.
Gastric inhibitory polypeptide (GIP)	Stimulates pancreatic secretion of insulin from normal B-cells.

These enteric hormones, and others, have a variety of additional effects that are unrelated to glucose metabolism and need not be mentioned here. It is important to remember that:

1. As a group, enteric hormones tend to cause BG to rise if B-cells are unable to produce sufficient insulin.

2. The secretion of enteric hormones is stimulated by the presence of food, or digestive processes in the stomach or

gut. Several are stimulated by physical distension of the gut, others by breakdown products of fat, carbohydrate, or protein digestion, and so on.

Thus any food entering the gut will stimulate a variety of enteric hormones, most of which will cause BG to increase, unless they are opposed by insulin. In the diabetic, there may be an absolute or a relative deficiency of insulin. As a result, even foods that cannot be broken down to glucose by digestion (for example, fats) will cause rapid BG elevation in many diabetics. In most cases these effects are trivial when small portions are eaten but can be very substantial during and after large meals.

6

THE DIFFERENT TYPES OF DIABETES MELLITUS

SUMMARY

Different types of diabetes require different approaches to treatment. C-peptide, a by-product of insulin manufactured by functioning B-cells, can be measured as an index of remaining insulin production. The urinary C-peptide level in a 24-hour collection can help the clinician determine which type of treatment is most appropriate. This measurement helps us distinguish between various types of insulin-dependent diabetes. The major classifications of diabetes may be broken down as follows:

Type I.   Insulin-Dependent Diabetes Mellitus (IDDM)

Injected insulin is required for the maintenance of life. These patients will benefit most from the GLUCOGRAF method. This category is further broken down into:

TYPE IA.   IDDM WITH NEGLIGIBLE C-PEPTIDE LEVELS

Includes the classic "juvenile onset" type of diabetes. Most patients in this subgroup respond to Regular insulin and to glucose loading with predictable BG responses that can often be duplicated from one patient to another.

TYPE IB.   **IDDM WITH SIGNIFICANT C-PEPTIDE LEVELS**

While still producing some endogenous insulin, these patients require supplementary doses of injected insulin. The BG response to Regular insulin and to glucose loading varies considerably from patient to patient. These patients therefore require highly customized treatment regimens.

Type II.   Non-Insulin-Dependent Diabetes (NIDDM)

Individuals in this group can survive without exogenous (injected) insulin, but some may require such insulin for the continuous maintenance of normal BG levels. There are two major subtypes within this category:

TYPE IIA.   **OBESE NIDDM**

Patients are more than 20 percent overweight and have deficiencies in insulin binding sites on target cells, stemming somehow from their obese condition. Their endogenous insulin thereby becomes relatively ineffective. The appropriate treatment usually includes weight reduction, frequently combined with other modes of therapy. Most diabetics fall into this category.

TYPE IIB.   **NONOBESE NIDDM**

These patients frequently have retarded phase I insulin release in response to meals, but produce adequate insulin to normalize BG when fasting. While many individuals in this group do well on special diets and numerous small daily meals, others may benefit from selected aspects of the GLUCOGRAF system.

IDDM and NIDDM During Pregnancy

Historically, the incidence of fetal and maternal morbidity, fetal mortality, and birth defects has been very high when the mother has been diabetic. These problems have been eliminated in studies where BG is normalized throughout pregnancy. The GLUCOGRAF regimen must undergo a number of modifications for treating IDDM during the prenatal and perinatal periods in order to meet the unique metabolic changes that occur during pregnancy.

Insulin-Resistant IDDM

There are two types of insulin resistance, immune and nonimmune. Both may require very large daily insulin usage. The guidelines for insulin dosage set forth in Chapter 12 will not apply to these cases and considerable experimentation may be required for the physician to develop a regimen that works for a given patient.

Pediatric IDDM

Results of applying the GLUCOGRAF method to pre-adolescents have not been reported (to our knowledge). Since so much of the regimen depends upon self-management by the patient, physicians have devoted their early efforts to more mature individuals. The special problems that may apply to the treatment of very young patients are probably more psychological than physiological, but have not yet been adequately explored.

Diabetes mellitus is a term that includes myriad diseases, all of which have the effect of impairing the ability of the body to transport glucose from the blood into cells where it can be used for immediate energy or converted to energy reserves.

In 1979, the National Diabetes Data Group of the National Institutes of Health proposed a list of types and subtypes of diabetes, based upon causative and other factors, to be used to coordinate terminology in clinical and epidemiological research.[1] I have chosen to utilize some of the major classifications of this proposal but have modified the types of diabetes to coincide more appropriately with the different approaches to treatment that are considered.

Type I.   Insulin-Dependent Diabetes Mellitus (IDDM)

Persons in this classification are dependent upon injected insulin to prevent the accumulation of toxic ketonic acids in their blood. In most cases, the bulk of the B-cells in the pancreas have been destroyed. Many of these patients require daily injections for the maintenance of life. Patients in this group can be helped by all facets of our regimen.[2]

We must, however, distinguish between two subclasses of IDDM patients: those with C-peptides and those without.

Figure 1 schematically illustrates the structure of a molecule of proinsulin—a protein precursor of insulin, produced inside the B-cells of the pancreas. (See page 48.) Proinsulin is converted into insulin by the removal of the curved part of the molecule designated "connecting peptide" (or C-peptide). C-peptide is released into the bloodstream at about the same time as insulin and excreted via the urine without performing any known function other than facilitating the folding of the insulin molecule. If a patient's pancreas is producing even a small amount of insulin, some C-peptide will be detectable by special blood and urine tests. It is highly desirable, but not essential, that patients be tested for the

---

1. National Diabetes Data Group. Classification and Diagnosis of Diabetes Mellitus and Other Categories of Glucose Intolerance, *Diabetes* 28:1039–1057 (1979).

2. This may be especially true for newly diagnosed patients, in the light of recent research indicating that early continuous normalization of BG *may possibly* prevent total loss of insulin production by the B-cells of the pancreas.

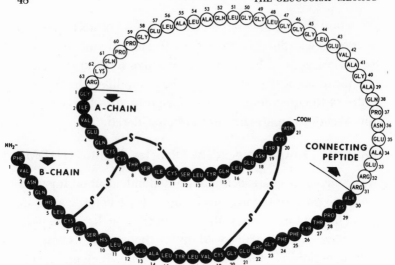

Figure 1. Removal of C-peptide (light circles) from proinsulin molecule leaves insulin molecule (dark circles). *Courtesy Eli Lilly and Company.*

C-peptide levels in a 24-hour urine collection before introduction to the GLUCOGRAF regimen, so that current levels of insulin production can be estimated. Normal values for this determination will probably vary from one laboratory to another. Clinical laboratory personnel or physicians can secure further information about this test from Bio-Science Laboratories, 7600 Tyrone Avenue, Van Nuys, California 91405.

Type Ia.   IDDM with Less than 5 Percent of Normal C-peptide Levels

Most of the patients in this subcategory become diabetic before they reach 40 years of age. Frequently onset occurs during childhood or adolescence ("juvenile onset"). Other patients become diabetic via surgical removal of or chemical injury to the pancreas and other rare causes. These patients produce very little or no endogenous (their own) insulin. It can be said that they have no glucose tolerance. If these patients are not given insulin by injection (exogenous), none of the insulin-requiring tissues will be able to utilize glucose, and nearly all dietary carbohydrate and protein will only serve to raise blood and urine glucose levels. Untreated patients will even have elevated BG while fasting, because they have no insulin to oppose the counter-regulatory hormones that cause gluconeogenesis and glycogenolysis (see Chapter 5).

Since, when untreated, their metabolic systems will be breaking down fats for fuel, ketones will appear in blood and urine. These patients are usually designated as "brittle" or "labile." These terms reflect the extreme or wild BG swings that such patients experience. It is not unheard of for an individual in this category to show BG values that swing from as low as 20 mg/dl to as high as 700 mg/dl, within a period of 1 hour. *Wild swings in BG are usually not due to the underlying disease but rather to an inappropriate approach to treatment.* Unfortunately, satisfactory treatment of this type of patient has, before the development of the GLUCOGRAF regimen, been extremely rare. Since this patient is not producing any endogenous insulin, his body cannot prevent the rapid rise in BG that occurs during a meal. He requires a very special diet and insulin program to get through meals without either a dramatic BG increase or hypoglycemia from improper use of insulin. If a type Ia patient is not pregnant, or obese, or growing, or producing high levels of insulin antibodies, he or she will typically require a *maximum* daily insulin dose, under the regimen, of about ½ unit per kilogram of body weight (¼ unit per pound). These individuals stand to benefit most from the GLUCOGRAF method, because their BG's are the most difficult to control by usual approaches. This manual is therefore particularly useful for this type of patient.

Type Ib.   IDDM with C-peptide Levels Greater than 5
                          Percent of Normal

Persons in this group are producing some endogenous insulin, but do not demonstrate enough effective insulin activity to allow them to live without daily injections. They are
less "brittle" than type Ia patients, in that their BG values
will usually not be found to swing as wildly. Furthermore,
they will require less injected insulin than will comparable
type Ia patients. Some of these Ib patients can continually
produce the small amounts of endogenous insulin necessary
to prevent gluconeogenesis, glycogenolysis, and lipolysis
while fasting but cannot put out the large phase I spurts of
insulin that are necessary during meals. Nevertheless, many
of these patients can, assisted by small amounts of exogenous
(injected) insulin, comfortably process meals with more carbohydrate content than can type Ia patients. Type Ib patients may also require a different range of calibrations
indicating the effects upon BG levels of administered doses
of insulin or glucose. Exogenous insulin is usually more effective in Ib patients because it is supplemented by their own
insulin. Similarly, in this group, carbohydrate usually has less
effect on BG, because increases in BG are partially compensated by release of endogenous insulin.

The rules for treatment of most type Ia patients will be
fairly rigid and nearly identical from one patient to the next,
because these patients are all in a similar situation—having
essentially no endogenous insulin.

Type Ib patients present more variability between individuals. One may be producing considerably more endogenous insulin than another and therefore significant
differences in treatment and response should be anticipated.

Type II.   Non-Insulin-Dependent Diabetes Mellitus (NIDDM)

Most people in this group become diabetic after age 40. These patients can survive without exogenous (injected) insulin and are not likely to produce ketones if untreated. Some members of this group, nevertheless, may be using insulin to control persistent BG elevation. In most cases, onset of glucose intolerance is not caused by destruction of B-cells. Descriptions of the two major subcategories of NIDDM follow.

Type IIa.   Obese NIDDM

The majority of diabetics fall into this subgroup. These patients exceed ideal body weight by at least 20 percent. Their diabetes appears to originate, not with a defect in insulin production, but rather with a deficit in the ability of insulin-dependent cells (muscle, fat, liver, etc.) to bind the insulin molecule to surface membranes. This deficit appears to be due to an inadequate number of insulin binding sites on the cell membranes. For reasons that are currently unclear, impaired insulin binding relates to obesity.[3]

In any event, the net result is elevated BG—usually postprandially (after meals) but sometimes also before meals. In response to the chronic elevation of BG, the B-cells produce

---

3. According to one theory, excess adipose tissue (body fat) somehow causes a reduction in insulin receptor sites at target tissues. The resulting BG elevation leads to exaggerated insulin production. The high tissue levels of insulin inhibit binding site formation, thereby rendering the insulin less effective for lowering BG. The further elevated BG causes even greater insulin production, and the cycle accelerates, eventually leading to B-cell exhaustion and IDDM. Another theory implicates reduced production of pancreatic polypeptide as the factor that initiates deactivation of insulin binding sites in obesity.

more and more insulin. In fact, insulin production can be considerably greater than normal in the early stages. This only serves to aggravate the condition, because increased blood insulin levels will result in a further reduction in availability of insulin binding sites.

The obvious treatment for this form of diabetes is weight reduction. Insulin therapy is usually contraindicated, because it can either cause further weight gain (see page 40) or further reduction in availability of binding sites. Our low-carbohydrate/high-protein diet is of possible value here, because it is less likely to cause precipitous postprandial BG elevation which would bring about even further overproduction of insulin.

If promptly treated by weight reduction, many cases of this type can be cured of overt glucose intolerance (diabetes). On the other hand, prolonged delay in treatment can possibly lead to irreversible loss of some B-cell function and a shifting of the patient to an IDDM category. Since the GLUCOGRAF regimen is concerned mostly with the use of injected insulin, in precisely controlling BG, it will be of lesser value to most obese NIDDM individuals.

Type IIb.   Nonobese NIDDM

A common defect in this type of diabetes is impaired phase I performance of the B-cell—that is, the initial release of insulin granules, in response to increased BG or other stimuli, is inadequate. Thus BG is usually elevated after meals. Eventually phase II production of insulin does reduce BG, possibly down to normal, before the next meal. The routine use of insulin in treating many of these patients is currently a matter of controversy. Our overall regimen is probably not applicable to most of these patients but some facets can be utilized in certain cases. For example:

1. Monitoring of BG by patients, and of glycosylated hemoglobin by physicians, may be warranted. In most cases, 6 daily BG measurements are not necessary if most after-meal (postprandial) determinations are in the normal range.

2. If the physician feels that, in a given patient, BG control can be facilitated by using insulin, then pre-meal (preprandial) doses of Regular insulin will probably give better results than will the usual one or two daily doses of intermediate-acting insulin. In these patients, it may be only the postprandial BG that is abnormal. Longer-acting insulins do not attack this problem.

3. There may be advantages to our high-protein/low-carbohydrate diet. It may even eliminate the need for supplementary insulin or oral hypoglycemic drugs. In some of these patients, however, a low CHO (carbohydrate) diet can work against the patient, by failing to provide the glucose challenge that keeps the B-cells producing insulin at a reasonable rate. Only repeated postprandial BG monitoring, over a period of weeks, will determine whether a given patient will respond better to a low CHO diet than to the widely prescribed high CHO diets.

IDDM During Pregnancy

Both IDDM and NIDDM may be precipitated by pregnancy, either as temporary or as permanent conditions. We will be concerned only with *IDDM* of pregnancy. If only temporary, it is called gestational IDDM. Alternately, an IDDM patient may become pregnant. Whatever the circumstances, IDDM during pregnancy can lead to increased infant morbidity and mortality, to birth defects, miscarriage, and serious complications in the mother (retinal hemorrhages, etc.), *if BG is not controlled meticulously from the onset of pregnancy.* Perhaps our regimen is most rewarding to both physician and patient when used during pregnancy. If used properly, among other benefits, it can eliminate the need for early delivery and cesarean section so commonplace in diabetic pregnancies.

An entire volume could be written on the modifications of the GLUCOGRAF method for use during pregnancy. Some major modifications may be summarized as follows:

1. Calibration of the effect of short-acting (Regular) insulin on BG will vary during the course of the pregnancy due mainly to changes in blood and tissue levels of various hormones.

2. Calibration of the effect of glucose tablets or sweets on BG for control of hypoglycemia will also vary as pregnancy proceeds.

3. The target BG level can be about 20 percent lower than in the nonpregnant patient because nondiabetics usually have lower BG when pregnant.

4. Hypoglycemia should be meticulously avoided as it can injure the fetus. This may require BG measurements every few hours.

5. Because the fetus has high carbohydrate requirements, it may be necessary to experimentally increase the dietary carbohydrate of the pregnant patient.

6. While our regimen calls for elimination of between-meal snacks, they are usually necessary to fill the continuous nutritional requirements of pregnancy. This may, in turn, necessitate additional small doses of Regular insulin.

7. At various times during pregnancy, there may be rapid changes in daily insulin requirements. Such changes are difficult to make on a day-to-day basis with basic long-acting insulin—Ultralente—because its effect on BG lasts several days. Therefore, it may be wise to treat pregnant IDDM patients with an intermediate-acting insulin (NPH), which is active for less than 24 hours. It is our experience that NPH is most effective if injected in 2 doses—exactly 12 hours apart.

In many patients this will mean that the evening dose of NPH must be administered several hours after the pre-evening-meal dose of Regular insulin, and therefore cannot be mixed with it. Thus, an additional injection may be required. In some people, a dose of NPH insulin will not even last 12 hours. For them, 3 doses of NPH, spaced 8 hours apart, may be necessary.

8. Because insulin requirements drop very rapidly, albeit briefly, after delivery, the dose of intermediate-acting insulin should be reduced 50 percent or more at onset of labor and for up to 2 weeks after delivery.[4] BG should be monitored every 3 hours during this period (at least hourly during labor), and supplementary small doses of Regular insulin or glucose tablets should be administered, in accordance with BG measurements. After this period, the dose of intermediate insulin should be determined experimentally. The patient should not be returned to long-acting insulin until about 2 weeks after delivery.

Insulin-Resistant IDDM

In rare cases, patients may require very large daily doses of insulin due to one of two types of insulin resistance: (1) immune resistance or (2) nonimmune resistance. In either type, requirements may range from less than 100 to 10,000 units per day. In one form of immune resistance, the body responds to small amounts of protein impurities in commercially prepared insulin by producing antibodies that react both with the injected impurities and with the injected insulin. Much of the insulin is thus rendered ineffective. Patients with this form of resistance are often treated successfully with monocomponent pork insulin, either alone or mixed with prednisone or with sulfated insulin (an investiga-

---

4. Some diabetic women whose pancreatic B-cells are still producing some insulin may require no insulin during labor.

tional drug manufactured by Connaught Laboratories, Toronto, Canada). In another form of immune resistance, antibodies to insulin receptors are produced. The receptors are blocked by the antibodies so that neither endogenous nor injected insulin can reach many of the receptor sites.

Nonimmune resistance can be due to the body's excessive production of counter-regulatory hormones. This sometimes implies the existence of abnormalities in one or more endocrine glands. Nonimmune resistance to insulin is not uncommon during the growth spurts of adolescence, and may be due to high blood levels of growth hormone, which has counter-regulatory effects. Deficiencies in insulin binding sites on target cells and "spilling" of insulin in the urine (renal wastage) constitute other forms of nonimmune resistance. Another type of nonimmune resistance involves enzymatic degradation of insulin at the site of subcutaneous injection. This can be circumvented by mixing the insulin with aprotinin (an enzyme inhibitor) or by injecting a number of small doses of Regular insulin into a vein every day.

Application of our regimen to insulin-resistant patients brings some added difficulty for the physician, because the simple calibrations of insulin effect on BG can vary greatly from one such patient to the next, and some of the dosage and timing guidelines set forth in Chapter 12 will not be applicable.

Pediatric IDDM

To our knowledge, results of using the GLUCOGRAF method in patients below 12 years of age have not been reported, although at least one pediatric diabetes center has young patients monitoring BG. This, as mentioned earlier, is because the technique is very new and clinicians feel that their early efforts will be more likely to succeed with patients who are emotionally and intellectually more mature.

Furthermore, grossly apparent diabetic complications are rarely encountered in preadolescent patients, so it has been said that these children have some time before physiologic BG control becomes mandatory. On the other hand, we know that the unpredictable wild swings in BG can cause considerable emotional turmoil and major psychological damage to youngsters. In addition, recent research indicates that sustained normalization of BG at onset of symptoms may preserve B-cell function in juvenile (type I) diabetes. Therefore a dilemma results that can be resolved only by careful clinical investigation in both the medical and psychological realms. At this point we cannot even suggest modifications of the regimen that might be appropriate for young patients.

7

PERTINENT BLOOD AND URINE TESTS

SUMMARY

1. 24-Hour Urinary C-peptide

Measured at the onset of treatment as an estimate of endogenous insulin production. This aids in classifying the patient for selection of approach to treatment.

2. Glycosylated Hemoglobin (Measured on Whole Blood)

Provides an estimate of the average blood sugar over the prior several weeks to 2 months. This may be the best test the physician has for evaluating degree of control. We urge that measurements be made prior to placing a patient on the GLUCOGRAF regimen and at least every 3 months thereafter.

3. Serum Lipids

Certain fat-related substances (lipids) found in the blood may be indirect indicators of: (A) predisposition to cardiovascular diseases; (B) changes in the degree of blood glucose control. Three different lipid measurements are discussed: triglycerides, total cholesterol, and HDL cholesterol.

There are several tests that can be performed on blood and urine which may be of considerable value to the physician in his efforts to assist the patient in maintaining normal BG and thereby remaining free from certain complications. It is important that the patient understand the significance of the various tests, as they can give him a gauge of the success of his own efforts. The blood or serum measurements listed in this chapter usually require several cubic centimeters (cc's) of blood, taken from a vein in the arm. These tests cannot be performed by the patient (as a BG measurement can) but require a clinical laboratory.

24-Hour Urinary C-Peptide Levels [1]

As already mentioned in Chapter 6, this test is a measure of the total daily production of endogenous insulin by the pancreatic B-cells. It helps the physician determine the classification of the patient's diabetes (types Ia, Ib, IIa, IIb, etc.). In general, the sequence of C-peptide levels runs approximately as shown in the following table.

Diagnostic Code	Designation	Usual 24-hour C-peptide (approximate) [2]
IIa	Obese NIDDM	Below normal to slightly above normal
IIb	Nonobese NIDDM	Below normal
Ib	IDDM, less labile	5 to 50 percent of normal
Ia	IDDM, more labile	None to 5 percent of normal

1. Urinary C-peptide determinations are not yet routinely available at many laboratories. Most university-affiliated medical centers and major commercial laboratories can measure serum C-peptide. Serum level, while not reflecting B-cell activity over an entire day, is an acceptable substitute for the urine measurement. For the serum test, a standard dose of oral glucose is first administered to the patient in an attempt to stimulate B-cells to release insulin.

2. At present, only a few studies of normal and diabetic 24-hour urinary C-peptide values have been published: see Appendix F, References 33, 36, 71. Normal values can be expected to vary considerably from one laboratory to another. Results are reported as micrograms per gram creatinine per day.

These broad classifications can be of considerable value to the physician in determining the initial form of treatment. Starting with the second void in the morning, the patient collects, in large bottles, all urine put out over the next 24 hours, up to and including the first void of the following morning. The urine must be kept under refrigeration until it is taken to the laboratory.

Glycosylated Hemoglobin—HbA$_1$ or HbA$_{1c}$—Measured on Whole Blood

Red blood cells (erythrocytes) contain a red pigment called hemoglobin. The hemoglobin molecule has a unique shape and other properties that enable it to pick up oxygen as blood passes through the lungs. The hemoglobin molecule later deposits the oxygen in body tissues, where it is essential for the normal cellular conversion of foodstuffs to energy (metabolism). Nearly all the hemoglobin in the normal adult exists in a form called hemoglobin A (HbA).

If a large number of erythrocytes are placed in a special nutrient solution containing glucose and maintained at body temperature, some of their hemoglobin A molecules will pick up glucose molecules. These glucose-binding hemoglobin molecules will be less efficient at releasing oxygen to tissues. At greater glucose concentrations, more hemoglobin molecules are so affected. The same process of glucose binding occurs in the bloodstream. The hemoglobin so produced is called glycosylated hemoglobin, or more precisely, hemoglobin A$_1$ (HbA$_1$). This HbA$_1$ can be measured in most clinical laboratories. It actually consists of four different molecular species, which differ from one another by several properties, including the site on the hemoglobin molecule that binds a glucose molecule. These four glycosylated hemoglobins are called HbA$_{1a1}$, HbA$_{1a2}$, HbA$_{1b}$, and HbA$_{1c}$. The HbA$_{1c}$ concentration is especially sensitive to changes in blood glucose concentration. It is less costly, however, for laboratories to measure total glycosylated hemoglobin (HbA$_1$) than to measure HbA$_{1c}$.

Since glycosylation continues throughout the life of a red cell, the measurement of HbA$_1$ or HbA$_{1c}$ will be related to the varying BG concentration over that lifetime. Since an erythrocyte lives in the body for about 4 months before it dies and is replaced, the average age of a sample of red cells is 2 months. Experiments indicate that the concentration of glycosylated hemoglobin in a patient's blood will correlate approximately with his average BG over the prior several weeks to 2 months, suggesting that young erythrocytes can incorporate more glucose than older ones.[3]

Nondiabetics usually have HbA$_{1c}$ values of perhaps 4–6 percent and HbA$_1$ values of perhaps 7–9 percent. In other words, 7–9 percent of their hemoglobin A molecules are glycosylated. Diabetic values of HbA$_{1c}$ have been measured as high as 22 percent, with typical values for IDDM of about 11 percent. Yet it is possible, and indeed expected, that on our regimen, even type Ia patients can have HbA$_{1c}$ values in the normal 4–6 percent range, or HbA$_1$ values in the 7–9 percent range. Actual values for normal ranges may vary from one laboratory to another.

The measurement of HbA$_{1c}$ or HbA$_1$ can be of value to the clinician in at least four ways:

1. It can be used as a double check on the BG reports presented by the patient. For example, if a patient measures BG six times daily, and reports all values as under 200 mg/dl for 2 months, HbA$_{1c}$ in the low end of the diabetic range (7–9 percent) might be expected. If the actual HbA$_{1c}$ is 12 percent, the patient may be measuring BG improperly or falsifying results.

3. Recent studies indicate that patients' red blood cells must be incubated in saline at 37°C. for 5 hours prior to measuring glycosylated Hb, to deglycosylate a rapidly formed labile species of HbA$_{1c}$ which reflects BG several hours prior. Clinicians should therefore be certain that their laboratories perform this incubation before relying on glycosylated Hb as an indicator of longer-term BG control.

2. Successive monthly or bimonthly measurements of glycosylated hemoglobin serve as a gauge of treatment progress. Improvements in average BG will be reflected in lowered values. These measurements provide a continuing incentive for the patient to comply with the program and to take the responsibility for his own well-being.

3. Many of the vascular (blood-vessel) complications of diabetes are related to the glycosylation of proteins in the walls of blood vessels. It is believed that abnormal glycosylation of many tissue proteins results from excessively high BG. Therefore, HbA_{1c} can serve as a crude indicator of the degree of jeopardy to which a patient is exposed if his current value remains unchanged for a number of years. On the other hand, consistently normal values of HbA_{1c}, year after year, should assure both the clinician and the patient that the hazards of complications are probably nonexistent.[4]

4. HbA_1 or HbA_{1c} levels can be used as diagnostic screening tests for unknown or suspected diabetes. They are less costly, less time consuming and less traumatic than the glucose tolerance test and do not require that the patient be fasting.

We advise that clinicians secure measurements *at least* every three months, and that a baseline value be secured before treatment under the new regimen begins. The continuing improvement in values is a measurable reward to both physician and patient for the hard work required during the first few weeks of treatment.

Serum Lipid Determinations

Lipids include a variety of chemical substances related to fats, with the properties of being insoluble or slightly soluble in water, but highly soluble in "non-polar" solvents like chlo-

---

4. Recent studies of diabetic patients, using the technique of quantitative vitreous fluorometry, for example, indicate that leakage of blood vessels, in the retina of the eye, drops from diabetic levels to nondiabetic levels (5.4 ± 0.3 ng/ml) as elevated HbA_{1c} drops to the normal range.

roform and ether. Because they have low solubility in water they are usually found in the blood bound to protein carriers called lipoproteins. Under certain conditions, they can leave the blood, by being deposited on the walls of blood vessels. These deposits can be a causative factor in diseases of the blood vessels (vascular diseases). Since uncontrolled diabetics usually have an abnormal predisposition to vascular disease and because serum levels of certain lipids, such as total and HDL cholesterol, may also be abnormal, there is usually interest in the patient's serum levels of these lipids.

Frequently serum levels of certain lipids are used by physicians as indicators of recent BG control. But since other factors than diabetes can affect the various lipid tests, *they are only positive indicators of BG control when compared to prior values for the same patient.*

Although glycosylated hemoglobin measurement is far more reliable as an indicator of BG control than are any of the lipid tests, this determination is not yet offered by hospital laboratories in some parts of the country. Furthermore, since abnormal values for certain lipid measurements correlate statistically with predisposition for cardiovascular (that is, heart and blood vessel) disease, the physician may wish to have the following blood lipid determinations performed periodically.

Serum Triglycerides

Triglycerides (more properly called triacylglycerols) are the principal type of fat stored by the body as reserve fuel. They can be manufactured in the liver from blood glucose. High BG level, especially in obese individuals, may elevate serum triglycerides in poorly controlled diabetes. Because dietary factors also affect their production, serum triglyceride levels are measured when the patient is fasting—that is, before breakfast. Until the HbA_{1c} test became routinely available, serum triglyceride values were used by some diabetologists as periodic crude indicators of recent BG control. Clinicians, however, encountered two problems:

1. Fasting measurements were inconvenient to patients.

2. Fasting triglyceride values could still vary considerably from day to day, albeit not as much as fasting BG, and therefore at best indicate recent degree of control rather than average control of BG over several weeks.

Serum triglyceride values are reported in milligrams of triglyceride per deciliter (1/10 liter) of serum (mg/dl). Approximate normal values for the general population are 50–150 mg/dl. Chronically elevated fasting triglyceride values are believed to increase the risk of cardiovascular disease.

Total Cholesterol

Another serum lipid that is usually elevated in poorly controlled diabetes, total cholesterol, also does not correlate with average BG as well as HbA_{1c}. It has the advantage over triglycerides of varying slowly over a period of several weeks. Fasting measurements are not necessary and values are also reported in mg/dl. Total cholesterol is a less accurate indicator of susceptibility to cardiovascular disease than the more modern HDL cholesterol, discussed later. Approximate normal values for the general population are in the range of 130–230 mg/dl, with levels for males tending to be higher than for females of the same age (up to age 60). Recently an international panel of cardiologists and nutritionists suggested that appropriate target ranges should be 130–160 mg/dl for adults and 120–140 mg/dl for children. Chronic elevation of serum cholesterol has been found to correlate with incidence of cardiovascular disease.

HDL Cholesterol

Cholesterol is carried in the blood bound to a variety of

lipoproteins which may be separated from one another in the laboratory, into fractions of differing densities. These fractions have been classified as high-density, low-density, and very low-density lipoproteins; abbreviated as HDL, LDL, and VLDL respectively. The portion of total cholesterol which is bound to high-density lipoproteins is called HDL cholesterol or simply HDL. People with coronary heart disease tend to have *lower* levels of serum HDL than unaffected individuals of the same age and sex. There are indications that poorly controlled diabetics also have low HDL levels. Normal values range from about 40 to 60 mg/dl for males and from about 45 to 75 mg/dl for females. Normal values will vary considerably from one lab to another. For diabetics, *changes* in HDL may be better indices of control than the absolute value.

Of all the blood tests described in this chapter, HbA_{1c} and HbA_1 are the most direct gauges of average BG control and should be used for this purpose in preference to the other tests. The various lipid tests are, nevertheless, valuable as gauges of cardiovascular risk. Additional tests, which measure early, hopefully reversible, diabetic complications, are mentioned in Chapter 17.

It is our philosophy that laboratory determinations should be shared with patients. This means giving patients photocopies of lab reports and honestly discussing all relevant results, whether favorable or unfavorable. This is only proper since the patient (or his insurer) has paid for the tests and the patient puts far more time and energy into the treatment of his disease than does the health care professional. We find that when the patient is thus regarded as a partner in his own care he is more likely to treat his disease in a responsible fashion.

8

EQUIPMENT FOR MEASURING BLOOD GLUCOSE

SUMMARY

Urine testing for insulin users is not only a poor indicator of BG level but can frequently show much sugar when BG is low and little sugar when BG is high. BG can be measured by the patient in one or two minutes using one drop of blood and disposable plastic "reagent strips" that change color. All of the currently available equipment and supplies for measuring BG are described and illustrated in this chapter. Cost information and addresses of suppliers are also given. Specific product recommendations are explained. These recommendations may be summarized as follows:

1. People who take insulin should use DEXTROSTIX® reagent strips, which must be read on the DEXTRO-METER™ or GLUCOMETER™ reflectance colorimeters (Ames Co.). They should own *two* rechargeable battery packs for powering the DEXTROMETER when away from home or two sets of four rechargeable AA batteries with charger for the GLUCOMETER. For emergency situations they should have on hand a vial of CHEMSTRIP® bG reagent strips (Bio-Dynamics/bmc, Division of Boehringer Mannheim) which can be used to estimate BG visually without a meter.

2. Patients who do not use insulin will find it more convenient to use the CHEMSTRIP bG reagent strips.

3. Many patients will find the following products helpful for pricking their fingers:

a. MONOLET® lancets (Sherwood Medical Industries).
b. AUTOLET® spring-driven lancet holder (Bio-Dynamics/bmc).

Although supplies for BG measurement can be costly, the entire regimen is actually a money-saver because normalization of BG can eliminate most hospitalizations and loss of earnings and can bring about a major reduction in food consumption.

For many years, insulin-dependent diabetics have been taught to monitor glucose in their urine and to use urine glucose level as a guide to insulin dose, diet, and exercise. Urine glucose was selected because, until very recently, the measurement of blood glucose was beyond the capability of patients.

When BG exceeds a certain concentration, called the renal (kidney) threshold,[1] a portion of the excess glucose is excreted or "spilled" into the urine by the kidneys. The renal threshold value of BG is usually in the range 150–180 mg/dl for the population at large. Unfortunately, individuals show considerable variations from one to another. Furthermore, the renal threshold for one person may vary over a period of weeks or months. Thus a patient cannot be certain of his BG at the moment he first begins to spill a trace amount of urine glucose. His efforts to estimate BG from urine sugar can be further confused by the fact that his urine test may show more glucose than just a trace. What BG value then corresponds to a given percent of urine glucose? This question cannot be answered because the concentration of urine glucose is determined by many factors in addition to BG. For example, fluid consumption will reduce urine glucose concentration. Furthermore, there is a limit to which the kidney

---

1. More correctly, when glucose concentration in the filtrate that the kidney removes from blood exceeds the kidney's ability to put glucose back into the blood (renal resorptive capacity).

can concentrate glucose in the urine. As a result, when BG exceeds a certain value the urine glucose concentration will no longer increase.

All of these sources of error are minor in comparison to the error that can be caused by the delay that occurs between an increase in BG and an increase in urine glucose or a decrease in BG and a decrease in urine glucose. This delay can vary in a given patient between ½ hour and 2 hours.[2] In a non-insulin-dependent, mild diabetic, who is well controlled by diet alone, and who rarely has an elevated BG, this is unimportant, since it is only the occasional urine that contains any glucose. But in the insulin-dependent patient who is using urine tests to adjust diet and insulin, this delay can be critical. It is just this type of patient who can show very rapid changes in BG. For example, after exercising, this patient may experience a sudden drop in BG to a very low level. If he tests his urine it may still show a high glucose level and deceive him into thinking that BG is still high. He might refrain from eating something sweet to raise his BG. He may then become mentally confused by the failure to provide his brain with urgently needed glucose, and unconsciousness can rapidly follow.

For the reasons stated, our regimen calls for the frequent direct measurement of BG by the patient. This can now be done simply and almost painlessly with blood obtained by a simple finger prick. At this point, the reader might wish to refer to Appendix C, page 248, for a summary of clinical studies of patients who measure BG in this fashion. However, some diabetics not requiring insulin are able to maintain normal BG 24 hours a day by strict dietary control. For such people, urines are always negative and urine testing may be used as an indicator of possible deterioration of the diabetic state. Certainly, urine testing can take the place of BG

---

2. It has been erroneously claimed that the "second void" method of urine testing circumvents this problem.

monitoring for these patients, provided that every few months HbA$_{1c}$ measurements are found to be absolutely normal.

The following equipment is now available from most surgical supply dealers for patients' use in measuring BG:

1. Plastic strips having a pad at one end that contains chemicals sensitive to glucose. One drop of blood is placed on this reagent strip and allowed to remain there for one minute. The blood is then removed from the strip which is read in an electronic instrument.

2. The electronic reading device is called a reflectance colorimeter. It converts the depth of color of the reagent strip to a number (BG value) which can be read on the face of the instrument.

Reagent Strips

At present, two different brands of reagent strips for use with reflectance colorimeters are available commercially:

1. DEXTROSTIX. Supplied in the U.S. by Ames Co., Division of Miles Laboratories, Inc., Elkhart, Ind. 46514. One minute is required for development of color. Blood must then be removed from the strip by a stream of ordinary tap water that the user squirts from a plastic squeeze bottle. (See Fig. 2, page 70.) Current retail cost in the U.S. is approximately $51.00 for a vial of 100 strips. Discount druggists are currently retailing DEXTROSTIX for about $41.00 per vial.[3]

2. StatTek test strips. Supplied in the U.S. by Bio-Dynamics/bmc, Division of Boehringer Mannheim, 9115 Hague Road, Indianapolis, Ind. 46250. These strips are marketed

---

3. Ames Co. has, in the U.S.A., designated certain distributors and medical centers as "Home Testing Centers." These centers not only stock Ames BG products but are supposedly capable of training patients in their use. Some of these centers are selling DEXTROSTIX and other Ames products at discounts. The names of nearby centers may be obtained by writing to the Ames Co.

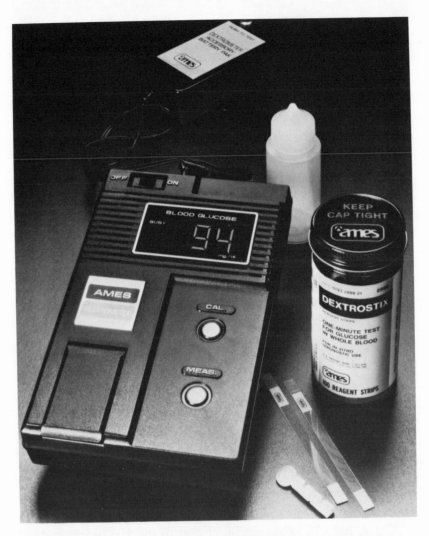

Figure 2. Ames DEXTROMETER digital readout reflectance colorimeter with rechargeable battery (rear). On the right are shown (from front to rear): a MONOLET lancet for pricking the finger (sealed to preserve sterility), two DEXTROSTIX reagent strips, a vial of 100 DEXTROSTIX, and a plastic squeeze bottle containing DEXTRO-CHEK standard glucose solution for calibrating the instrument. *Courtesy of Ames Co.*

outside the U.S. as "Reflomat glucose strips." Although two minutes are required for development of color, the blood may be removed from the strip by simply wiping with a

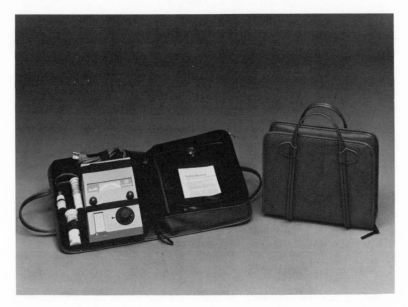

Figure 3. StatTek twin-beam reflectance photometer in carrying case (available from manufacturer). At far left, vial of StatTek reagent strips, and supplies for calibrating the instrument. *Courtesy of Bio-Dynamics/bmc.*

piece of cotton or soft cleansing tissue after the first minute; no water supply is required. (See Fig. 3.) Current retail cost in the U.S. is approximately $60.00 for a kit that contains materials for 100 tests.

A third reagent strip is available, designed to be read by eye, without the aid of a colorimeter. Called CHEMSTRIP bG in the U.S. (Haemo Glukotest® outside the U.S.) and supplied by the makers of StatTek, this strip has a two-color reagent pad that facilitates visual comparison with a color chart printed on the container (see Fig. 4, page 73). It has an accuracy of about plus-or-minus 10–20 percent throughout the normal range of BG values but can be grossly misread by a patient suffering from the mental confusion or visual disturbances that frequently accompany hypoglycemia. Current retail cost in the U.S.A. is approximately $13.00 for a vial of 25 strips (53 cents per test).

Reflectance Colorimeters

At present, six different reflectance colorimeters are being produced: [4]

1. GLUCO-CHEK. Supplied by Medistron Ltd., Alpine Works, Oak Road, Southgate Crawley, Sussex RH118AJ, England. (See Fig. 5, page 74.) Rechargeable battery. Pocket size. Current retail cost is approximately £91 ($180).

2. HYPO-COUNT. Supplied by Hypoguard, Ltd., 49 Grimston Lane, Trimley, Ipswich, Suffolk, IP10OSA, England. (See Fig. 6, page 75.) Rechargeable battery or line operated. For table top use.

3. R.A.H.C. GLUCOSE TESTER. Supplied by Australian BIO Transducers, P.O. Box 365, Dee Why, N.S.W. 2099, Australia. May be powered by line cord or by five "C" batteries. (See Fig. 7, page 76.) This instrument is currently sold only in Australia, by the father of a young diabetic. Its price is 95 Australian dollars.

The three preceding instruments share a major shortcoming, in that they cannot be internally calibrated by the user for differences in operator technique and for differences in sensitivity between one batch of reagent strips and the next. This can lead to significant reading errors that are beyond the control of the user. The readout display of all three meters is in European BG units (millimoles per liter—mmol/L) and must be multiplied by 18 to convert BG readings to the units used in the U.S.A. (mg/dl). At present, these meters can only be used with DEXTROSTIX—not with StatTek reagent strips, although a GLUCO-CHEK model for StatTek strips is in development. These instruments are not available in the U.S., but may be procured from friends living abroad.

---

4. Meters sold in the U.S. display BG as mg/dl. Those sold in Europe usually display BG as mmol/L (millimoles per liter) following the convention of most countries.

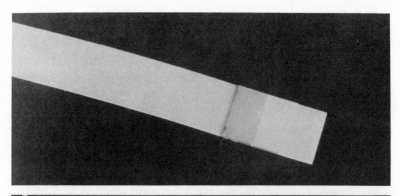

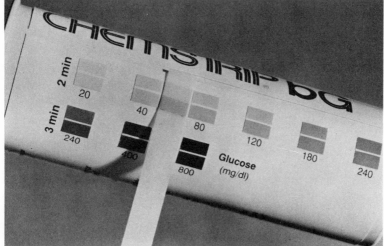

Figure 4. CHEMSTRIP bG reagent strips with two-color pad for estimating blood glucose visually. *Courtesy of Bio-Dynamics/ bmc.*

4. Ames DEXTROMETER. Same supplier as DEXTRO-STIX (see Fig. 2). This reflectance colorimeter digitally displays BG readings via light-emitting diodes. It measures 6¼ inches deep, 3⅞ inches wide, and 1½ inches high and weighs 13½ ounces with its rechargeable battery. Although too large for a pocket, it can be carried in a small shoulder bag (see Fig. 8, page 76) or in a somewhat larger carrying case available from the manufacturer. The DEXTROMETER can only be used with DEXTROSTIX. It currently retails for $340.00.

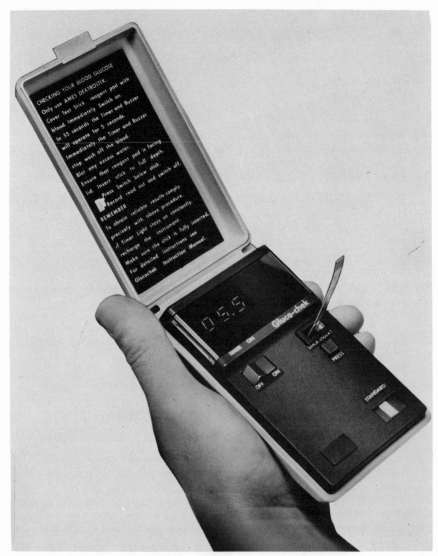

Figure 5. GLUCO-CHEK, reflectance colorimeter, containing rechargeable battery. *Courtesy of Medistron, Ltd.*

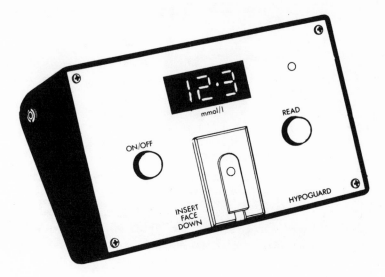

Figure 6. HYPO-COUNT, battery- or line-operated reflectance colorimeter. *Courtesy of Hypogaurd, Ltd.*

The rechargeable battery pack costs $35.00. A carrying case with shoulder strap is available for $40.00. On occasion a dealer can be found who will supply it at a discounted price.

5. Ames GLUCOMETER. Same supplier as DEXTRO-STIX and DEXTROMETER (see Fig. 9, page 78). This instrument measures 3¼ inches deep, 6⅝ inches wide, and 1-5/16 inches high. It weighs 12 ounces with 4 size AA batteries and can be carried in an overcoat pocket, a purse, or a small shoulder bag. The GLUCOMETER utilizes a liquid crystal digital display and a built-in timer and buzzer. It possesses a very important feature in that it can store calibrations after it has been turned off. The significance of this is discussed later in this chapter. The GLUCOMETER can only be used with DEXTROSTIX. At present (early 1981), it is only for sale in England and therefore is only available with BG readout in mmol/L (see footnote 4, on page 72). It

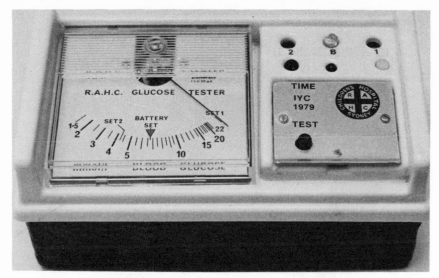

Figure 7. R.A.H.C. GLUCOSE TESTER —battery- or line-operated reflectance colorimeter. *Courtesy of Australian BIO Transducers.*

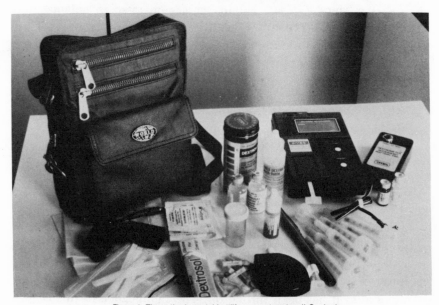

Figure 8. The author's portable "life support system." Contents of the shoulder bag include an Ames DEXTROMETER with rechargeable battery, a spare rechargeable battery, a plastic rinse bottle, an empty plastic vial (for receiving the rinse water), 1 vial each of insulin and glucagon, DEXTROSTIX, disposable insulin syringes, alcohol swabs, glucose tablets (DEXTROSOL), pen, AUTOLET lancet holder, MONOLET sterile disposable lancets, DEXTRO-CHEK glucose standard, paper napkins for blotting the DEXTROSTIX, a GLUCOGRAF data sheet (see Chapter 10) and a few CHEMSTRIP bG reagent strips (for use in buses and trains).

retails for £91 ($180) with 4 alkaline batteries. We suspect that the GLUCOMETER will become available in the U.S. and Canada (with mg/dl readout) during 1982.

6. StatTek twin-beam reflectance colorimeter (REFLO-MAT outside the U.S. and Canada). (See Fig. 3.) Same supplier as StatTek or REFLOMAT reagent strips. Although available with a satchel-size carrying case, this instrument cannot be battery-operated. Furthermore, its price ($675 with case) places it beyond most pocketbooks. This instrument was designed for use by clinical laboratories and can serve for other blood chemistry determinations in addition to glucose.

Finger-Pricking Equipment

1. MONOLET sterile disposable lancets. Manufactured in the U.S.A. by Sherwood Medical Industries, Inc., 1831 Olive Street, St. Louis, Mo. 63103. (See Figs. 2, 8, 10.) Although many other brands of disposable lancets are available, the MONOLET product produces very tiny punctures and is therefore the only one we recommend. Current retail price is $7.50 for a box of 200 lancets. Although sold as a disposable product, the lancet can be wiped with an alcohol sponge after each use, and the twist-off plastic cap replaced. The author reuses each lancet many times.

2. AUTOLET spring-driven lancet holder. Manufactured in England by Owen Mumford, Ltd., Oxford; distributed in the U.S. by Ulster Scientific, Inc., P.O. Box 902, Highland, N.Y. 12528. Also marketed by Bio-Dynamics/bmc and by Ames Co. (addresses given earlier). (See Fig. 10, page 79.) This compact, plastic device is a must for people who have never pricked their fingers before. It is not only a substitute for courage but, when used properly, can reduce the pain of a finger prick to virtually zero. Current retail price is about $25 in the U.S. The unit is designed for use with MONOLET lancets only.

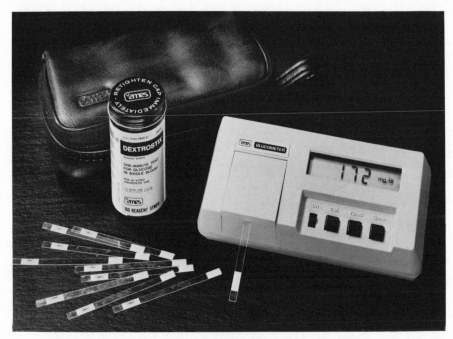

Figure 9. Ames GLUCOMETER digital readout reflectance color-imeter with built-in timer. For use with four size AA alkaline or rechargeable batteries.

3. Disposable hypodermic needles (30 gauge). Many people find that the 30-gauge (very fine) hypodermic needle provides a nearly painless finger stick. This is also the author's observation. Hypodermic needles, however, can penetrate the finger quite deeply if used carelessly. Many of us have plunged a ½-inch needle halfway into a finger. The result is usually a shriek, enough blood for 10 BG measurements, and a black and blue spot that lasts a week. The MONOLET lancet, while not as fine as a 30-gauge needle, has a point length of only ⅛ inch. If used properly it will penetrate less than half its length. Disposable hypodermic needles, 30 gauge, ½ inch, sell in the U.S. for about $25 for 100 needles, or 25 cents each. They come with plastic covers and can be reused if wiped with alcohol. They must be specially ordered

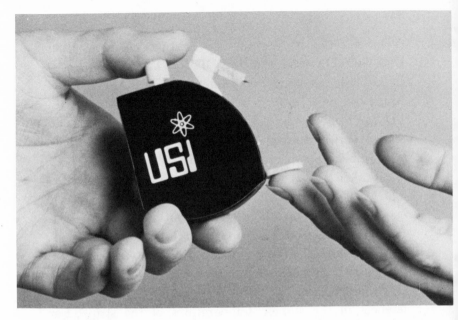

Figure 10. AUTOLET spring-driven holder for MONOLET lancets. Virtually painless if used properly. *Courtesy of Ulster Scientific, Inc.*

by the druggist but usually can be obtained within a few days. More readily available are 27-gauge needles, which cost less than half as much but are not as fine. Most disposable insulin syringes come with 27-gauge needles.

Recommended Equipment

Three different reagent strips and six different reflectance colorimeters have been listed here. This leaves the reader in a dilemma similar to that of the consumer who wants to buy his first camera or stereo system and must select among myriad brands and budgets. However, I consider that at the present time, only two combinations of instrument and reagent strips are really suitable for patients' use.

First, I reiterate that for finger pricking, we highly recommend the AUTOLET used with MONOLET lancets. The AUTOLET will be "virtually painless" only if used according to the method described in Chapter 9. If not used properly, it can do more harm than good.

Our selection of reagent strips narrows down to either DEXTROSTIX used with the DEXTROMETER or GLUCOMETER reflectance colorimeters or CHEMSTRIP bG which can only be read by eye. The StatTek strips (REFLOMAT outside the U.S.) at present can be used only with a large, very expensive reflectance colorimeter (see Fig. 3), which cannot be operated by battery.

All other reflectance colorimeters other than the DEXTROMETER and GLUCOMETER must be ruled out because they cannot be calibrated for variations in sensitivity of DEXTROSTIX from one production lot to the next. Contrary to what a sales representative may want you to believe, these variations can be very significant clinically. Furthermore, these variations can become greater as a result of differences in the storage temperatures of the strips. For example, if a dealer stores DEXTROSTIX near a steam pipe there will probably be a major reduction in sensitivity. Another variation is due to differences in technique from one user to the next. Accurate timing, for example, is important. One user may start timing his one minute early and finish the one minute late. Some users squirt on too much water, others use drops of blood that are too small. If a user consistently makes the same error this, as well as other variations, can often be offset by properly calibrating his vial of strips according to the methods described in Chapter 9.

Now, how to decide between CHEMSTRIP bG read by eye and DEXTROSTIX used with the DEXTROMETER or GLUCOMETER? The selection is very simple:

A. Patients using insulin should use the DEXTROSTIX/ DEXTROMETER or GLUCOMETER combinations unless they cannot possibly afford to purchase a meter or cannot master the simple techniques for operating the instrument (see Chapter 9). There are several reasons for this preference; three of the most important follow:

1. During attacks of hypoglycemia it is not uncommon for patients to completely lose the ability to read CHEMSTRIP bG strips visually, while still being fully capable of operating the DEXTROMETER or GLUCOMETER and securing an accurate reading.

2. The difference in cost between CHEMSTRIP bG (discount price about 52 cents each) and DEXTROSTIX (discount price about 41 cents each) should pay for a DEXTROMETER in less than two years or a GLUCOMETER in less than one year.

3. Accuracy in the use of CHEMSTRIP bG requires skill in interpolation—the process of estimating the exact location of color intensity between the values printed on the vial (see Fig. 4). This skill can be acquired but cannot be guaranteed. Furthermore, while CHEMSTRIP bG is more resistant to deterioration than DEXTROSTIX, when exposed to conditions of high humidity, there is no system of user calibration that can assure the accuracy of CHEMSTRIP as can be done with DEXTROSTIX.

B. Patients who use insulin should always have a supply of CHEMSTRIP bG on hand for emergencies. Emergencies can entail anything from meter failure (rare) to extended camping trips in localities where there is no power for recharging the battery. In any event, *owners of the DEXTROMETER should purchase two rechargeable battery packs.* One should be charging while the other is in use, so that there is always an emergency backup. Similarly, owners of the GLUCOMETER should purchase 8 rechargeable AA nickel cadmium batteries and one four-place battery charger at a photo or electronics store. Four batteries can power the meter while the other four are charging.

C. Patients who do not use insulin need not be bothered with a DEXTROSTIX/DEXTROMETER or GLUCOMETER system but should certainly measure blood glucose anywhere from several times per day to several times per month (if it remains in the range of 70–140 mg/dl). These patients will find CHEMSTRIP bG more convenient.

If at some time in the future both the GLUCOMETER and DEXTROMETER are sold in the same countries,[5] the GLUCOMETER would probably be the preferred instrument for patient use. Some reasons for this are:

a. The GLUCOMETER with enclosed batteries is considerably more compact than the DEXTROMETER with its external battery pack.
b. The GLUCOMETER has such a low power drain that battery life between charges is many times that of the DEXTROMETER.
c. The GLUCOMETER can be user-calibrated at two BG values versus one calibration point for the DEXTROMETER. This will improve accuracy over a wider BG range.
d. The GLUCOMETER, once calibrated, retains its calibrations for many days. The DEXTROMETER drifts continually and therefore must be calibrated prior to every use. Initial preparation of special calibration strips for the DEXTROMETER requires considerable time and effort.
e. The GLUCOMETER retains its calibration even after the meter has been turned off. Since the DEXTROMETER has considerable battery drain, the instrument must be turned off after each use and then recalibrated using our simplified procedure.

---

5. With appropriate readout units for the respective countries—mg/dl or mmol/L.

Another Look at Costs

The cost of equipment and reagent strips is still high for many patients. Negotiations with dealers can sometimes result in up to a 15 percent discount from list prices. In the U.S., however, instruments and reagent strips are covered by major medical insurance,[6] if prescribed by a physician. In several countries, the entire cost of reagent strips and sometimes of meters is borne by the government. There is rumor of possible future reductions in the prices of reagent strips sold to patients.

In spite of the current high cost, our system should still be "cost effective" because of the resultant improvement in patient health. In the U.S., diabetics spend, on average, one week every four years in the hospital (for treatment of avoidable complications), at an average cost of about $200 per day. Nearly all diabetes-related hospitalizations can be eliminated if BG is continually in or near the normal range. Many other expenses related to diabetic complications, such as surgery, professional fees, drugs, tests, etc., can obviously be eliminated if the complications are prevented from occurring. The loss of wages resulting from temporary or permanent disability is also avoidable.

Cost of supplies is also offset by the tremendous reduction in food consumption that many patients on our regimen experience. Poorly controlled diabetics lose calories, vitamins, and minerals in their urine. They are frequently hungry and often eat double the daily amounts consumed by their nondiabetic counterparts.

---

6. It would be wise for every family with a history of diabetes in a close relative to secure major medical insurance before the disease strikes. Most companies will not insure diabetics who were not insured prior to onset.

9

PATIENT SELF-MONITORING OF BLOOD GLUCOSE

SUMMARY

There is much to be learned about blood glucose measurement that is not covered by the instructions provided with the equipment and supplies described in Chapter 8. This chapter lists a number of essential shortcuts and tips that should assure both accuracy and convenience when measuring BG. This chapter should be read even by people who have already become veterans at BG monitoring.

The topics covered include:

1. Using the AUTOLET with MONOLET lancets to painlessly secure one drop of fingertip blood.
2. Timing the test.
3. Special precautions when using CHEMSTRIP bG.
4. Special precautions when using DEXTROSTIX.
5. Using the Ames GLUCOMETER reflectance colorimeter.
6. When to monitor blood glucose—and why.
7. Differences between laboratory and patient BG measurements.

This chapter covers in detail the technique of performing a finger puncture and gives some important hints on the use of the materials recommended in Chapter 8. It does not attempt to duplicate instructions already supplied by the manufacturers but supplements them with additional information and assesses inappropriate directions that certain manufacturers have included in their instruction booklets. This will be followed by detailed instruction as to when BG measurements should be performed.

The bulk of the chapter, relating to equipment, assumes that the user has on hand the products described and is familiar with the operating instructions supplied by the manufacturer. If this is not the case, the first eight sections will be difficult to understand and the reader may wish to skip directly to the section entitled "When to Monitor Blood Glucose—and Why" on page 91. Be sure to return to the beginning of this chapter when the equipment is on hand, as the following guidelines are very important.

Using the Autolet with Monolet Lancets to Secure Painlessly One Drop of Fingertip Blood

1. Select a finger. Thumb and little finger are preferred by many people because they tend to bleed more freely, but any finger will do.

2. If the finger is not clean, wash it. If it is cold, hold the entire hand under warm (not hot) water for about 15 seconds. A warm finger bleeds more readily than a cold one.

3. Insert a plastic platform into the AUTOLET, if one has not already been installed. Although the manufacturer has been shipping a number of extra platforms with each AUTOLET, they need not be discarded after each use unless the instrument is used on different people (to prevent transmission of blood-borne infections from one person to another).

4. Insert a MONOLET lancet in the arm of the AUTOLET and cock the AUTOLET.

5. Clean the fingertip thoroughly with alcohol (preceded by soap and water if it is visibly soiled), being sure to dry it off afterward.

6. Place the hole in the AUTOLET platform over the site on the finger that you wish to puncture. Patients initially prefer the periphery of the fingertip because it is usually less sensitive (see Fig. 10, page 79, and Fig. 11, page 88).

7. A less courageous individual can partially numb the fingertip by pressing it hard with an opposing digit during the prick, as shown in Figure 12 (page 88).

8. Now comes the trick that can make finger sticking truly painless. The pressure of the plastic platform on the fingertip is what determines how deeply the lancet point will penetrate. A heavily calloused adult thumb will require much more pressure than a child's little finger. You will discover that different fingers on the same hand require different pressures. The aim is to penetrate deeply enough to draw blood but not enough to cause pain. First press the finger very gingerly against the platform. Depress the release button. The lancet will come down but will probably not prick the finger. Repeat the procedure several times, each time increasing the pressure of the fingertip on the plastic platform. Eventually you will be using enough pressure to draw blood but probably not so much as to cause pain. After a week of measuring BG, you will know what the proper pressure is for each of your fingers.

9. If you've made a deep enough puncture, blood will flow freely from the site when you gently squeeze the fingertip. Squeeze until there is one large drop on the finger—enough blood to flood the reagent pad on the test strip. Sooner or later someone may advise you to wipe off the first drop of blood because it contains "tissue fluid." This is nonsense. The first drop will give the same BG reading as the second drop, if your technique is consistent.

10. Now invert the finger so that the blood hangs from the tip. Touch the drop to the reagent pad on a DEXTROSTIX or a CHEMSTRIP bG. The blood should transfer to the re-

agent pad, flooding it.

11. After you have become "professional" at drawing blood from the periphery of the fingers, try pricking the central region of the fingertip. Even though this region is more sensitive, your professional technique can make the prick painless. It just takes practice and the fine control provided by the AUTOLET.

Timing the Test

Timing is best done with a watch having a large-sweep second hand or with the built-in timer if the GLUCOMETER is used. A stopwatch is unnecessary and pushing the buttons can add unmeasured delay to the timing. Keep your eye on the second hand as you are about to transfer the drop of blood to the reagent strip. When contact is made, observe the time (in seconds, of course) and remember it. Put the strip down on a table or sink and wait out the one minute. If you, like the author, are likely to forget the starting time, write it down. I have a "magic slate" glued to the bathroom wall for this purpose. Memory can play tricks on you if BG is even slightly low.

Special Precautions When Using CHEMSTRIP bG

1. The reagent pad is coated with an invisible dialyzing membrane. The pores in this membrane can be clogged by oils from the skin, so don't handle the reagent pad.

2. At the time of this writing, all CHEMSTRIP bG test strips are supplied warped, so that they do not lie flat on a table. This can cause the drop of blood to slide off the reagent pad. This problem can easily be corrected by the user before applying any blood. Put the strip on a table top with the reagent pad facing down. Pull it across the edge of the table while pressing the strip against the edge with a finger. This

technique, which can also be used to straighten curled pho-
tographs, is very effective.

3. Do not wipe off blood with rough tissues as they might
strip off the dialyzing membrane. Soft cleansing tissues or
cotton are satisfactory.

Special Precautions When Using DEXTROSTIX

1. A plastic squeeze bottle, such as that supplied by the
manufacturer of the reagent strips, should be used to wash
blood from the reagent strip. Running tap water does not
usually have adequate velocity for rapid, complete removal
of blood. It is wise to have several squeeze bottles on hand
since sooner or later they are likely to be lost. Ames Co. has
been supplying a tiny squeeze bottle with the DEXTROME-
TER but not with the GLUCOMETER. Request at least one
large squeeze bottle for home use and several small squeeze
bottles for travel.

2. When washing blood from the strip, rest the untreated
side against the vertical inside surface of a tumbler or sink, so
that it is restrained from flopping back and forth in the
stream of water (see Fig. 13).

3. After color development, washing, and blotting, the
treated surface of the strip should be uniform in color.
Blotches or mottling indicate improper technique and incorrect results. Uneven color is usually due to one of the following causes:

a. Not enough blood was placed on the reagent pad; as a
   result, the blood dried along the edges of the pad.
b. Water was squirted on the reagent pad in too sharp a
   stream or it was concentrated on one spot, so that some
   of the blue dye was washed off the pad. This problem is
   most common when BG is high. As a result, DEX-
   TROSTIX may show a very high BG as lower than it
   really is.
4. The label on the DEXTROSTIX vial contains a color

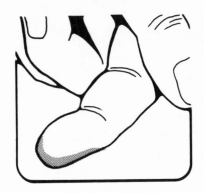

Figure 11. Since the periphery of the fingertip (shaded area) is usually less sensitive to pain, people initially prefer to puncture there.

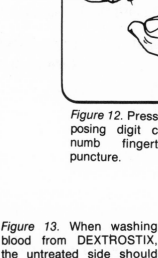

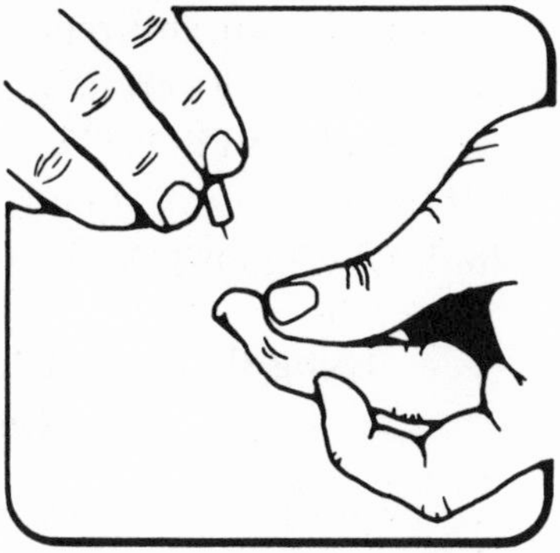

Figure 12. Pressure from opposing digit can partially numb fingertip during puncture.

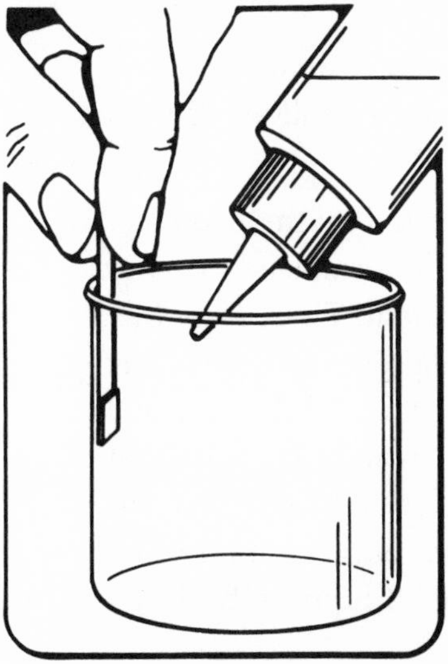

Figure 13. When washing blood from DEXTROSTIX, the untreated side should rest against the vertical inside surface of a tumbler or sink, so that it is restrained from flopping back and forth in the stream of water.

chart that supposedly can be used for estimating BG if reading an unblotted DEXTROSTIX without a meter. This chart should not be relied upon. The colors of the printing inks are very different from the colors that appear on the reagent pad and the inks are not changed with each production lot as they are on the vial of CHEMSTRIP bG. The color chart is of major value when an unconscious diabetic arrives at a hospital emergency room and the staff wants to determine if this individual's BG is very high (diabetic coma) or very low (hypoglycemia). Don't think that the chart can substitute for a meter in day-to-day management of BG.

5. In subfreezing climates, boats, camping vehicles, ski lodges and the like may have tap water systems that are protected with antifreeze mixtures. DEXTROSTIX reacts with traces of a certain antifreeze as if it were glucose. Do not rinse DEXTROSTIX with water suspected of containing antifreeze unless a drop of the water has been tested on a fresh DEXTROSTIX and has not caused a color change.

Using the Ames GLUCOMETER Reflectance Colorimeter

This instrument is virtually foolproof and should perform well if the manufacturer's instructions are followed, with three exceptions:

1. The two gray plastic sticks suggested by the manufacturer for an optional calibration procedure can lead to major errors if used for calibrating the instrument. There is no way that these two permanent standards can represent the colors of the reagent strips at 50 mg/dl (2.8 mmol/L) and 300 mg/dl (16.7 mmol/L) respectively when every batch of reagent strips is different and when every user performs his test somewhat differently. Therefore only calibrate the meter with the 50 mg/dl and 300 mg/dl liquid DEXTRO-CHEK calibrators.

2. The gray plastic sticks can, however, be used to check for drifting of the GLUCOMETER calibration when the instrument is used at a room temperature different from the temperature at the time of calibration. The plastic sticks can also be used to circumvent the need for daily "control tests." We suggest the following procedure for checking the instrument for drift.

Immediately after using the liquid DEXTRO-CHEK to

calibrate the meter for new batteries or for a new vial of DEXTROSTIX, etc., secure a reading on the light gray stick. Write this reading on the vial of DEXTROSTIX. Whenever the meter is turned on, its calibration can be rechecked by reading the light gray stick again. If the reading differs from the number written on the DEXTROSTIX vial by more than 5 percent, the instrument should be recalibrated using the *liquid* DEXTRO-CHEK calibrators.

3. Recalibrate the meter once every week even if it has not drifted. The meter may be fine but the DEXTROSTIX in your opened vial have aged somewhat and may have lost some of their sensitivity due to exposure to heat or humidity. Therefore be certain to recalibrate with the DEXTRO-CHEK calibrator glucose solutions.

Be sure to observe the precautions suggested in item 3 with regard to care of the vials of glucose solution.

When to Monitor Blood Glucose—And Why

We are now at a point where the patient can take the first step in his efforts to normalize BG. This step entails merely measuring and recording BG, *at least* six times daily, for a period of one to two weeks. The primary purpose of this introductory period is for the patient to become skilled in the rapid and accurate use of his new equipment. Another purpose is to demonstrate, to both physician and patient, the wide range of daily BG fluctuations that the patient usually experiences. There is no more graphic illustration of the need for corrective measures. The resulting awareness will be the major incentive for strict adherence to the new regimen.

During the introductory period, the patient should also record urine glucose levels at every void. The purpose of this is to demonstrate clearly to the patient that urine glucose is a very poor indicator of BG and to thereby justify the termination of reliance upon urine tests. Upon completion of the introductory phase, urine need no longer be tested.

BG should be recorded daily, by the patient, according to the following schedule:

1. Upon arising in the morning.
2. 2–3 hours after breakfast.
3. 1½ hours prior to midday meal.
4. 2–3 hours after midday meal.
5. 1½ hours prior to evening meal.
6. 2–3 hours after evening meal.
7. Immediately before retiring for the night.

BG should also be measured:

1. At the first suspicion of hypoglycemia (insulin reaction) and 2 hours after subsequent treatment to raise BG (see Chapter 14).

2. Prior to every snack and, where feasible, two hours thereafter. (This will be discontinued later, when the patient eliminates regular snacks.)

3. Before and after exercising.

The second group of measurements will frequently be made at the time designated for a BG measurement in the first group, so that the total number of measurements in a day will usually not exceed 8, once snacks have been discontinued.

All BG measurements should be recorded by the patient on a GLUCOGRAF form. A copy of the form suitable for photocopying and instructions for record keeping appear in the following chapter.

Examination of this BG schedule shows that it is designed to measure the effect that meals, snacks, exercise, etc., have on BG. It would be impossible to gauge the effect of breakfast on BG unless we measure both before and after eating. The 2–3 hour postprandial (after-eating) delay allows time for dietary protein and complex carbohydrate to be broken down to glucose in the digestive process.

The measurement of BG during and 2 hours after hypoglycemic attacks will frequently bring some surprises. Many patients will observe that hypoglycemic symptoms, such as hunger, nervousness, tachycardia (rapid heart rate), etc., frequently occur at normal or elevated BG, and therefore do not represent real hypoglycemia. Since most patients consume excessive carbohydrates for treatment of hypoglycemia, they will frequently observe excessive BG elevation 2 hours thereafter. With the help of these measurements the patient will learn (see Chapter 14) how to prevent this improper rebound of BG.

Once the patient has converted his diet and insulin dosage to the new regimen, the purpose of the BG monitoring will be, initially, to help "fine tune" diet and insulin for the maintenance of normal BG. Thereafter, it will serve to permit rapid correction of even slightly high or low BG, before the deviations proceed to a point where correction is difficult. Variance from ideal BG will be inevitable, even under the GLUCOGRAF regimen. Some of the reasons for this are:

1. The site of insulin injection (arm, hip, thigh, abdomen) affects the rate of absorption.

2. Physical activity will vary from day to day.

3. Meal portions will not be weighed or measured precisely, so there will be some variation in protein and carbohydrate intake.

4. The timing of insulin administration, prior to a meal, may vary because of unexpected delays and the like.

5. Illness, physical and extreme emotional stress, certain drugs, and menstrual cycle all affect the body's release of counter-regulatory hormones.

For practical purposes we will consider "ideal" BG as 100 mg/dl. This is the midpoint of our so-called normal range of perhaps 80–120 mg/dl. This ideal BG is for target purposes only. Any corrections of BG (see Chapters 12 and 14) will be directed toward this 100 mg/dl target. When BG measurements equal or exceed 120 mg/dl or are equal to or lower than 80 mg/dl, certain corrective measures will be taken— hopefully before BG strays much outside the 80–120 mg/dl range.

Differences Between Laboratory and Patient BG Measurements

Attempts to correlate BG measured by patients with BG measured by a professional laboratory will sometimes show differences. This is due to two effects:

1. The patient will be measuring *whole blood* glucose, while most clinical laboratories first discard the blood cells and clotted material and measure *serum* glucose. This difference causes our method to give a lower reading.

2. Clinical laboratories usually use venous (vein) blood, while our method uses arterial (capillary) blood. After a meal, arterial blood contains more glucose, some of which is delivered to body tissues, before the blood is returned to the heart via the venous system. This effect causes our method to read higher.

The effects mentioned approximately cancel one another after a meal. Our preprandial values, with the DEXTRO- STIX system, may be as much as 20 percent lower than those of many clinical laboratories. In order to avoid confusing the patient, we usually advise that treatment be based upon un- corrected meter readings that are not adjusted to compensate for the use of capillary whole blood, instead of serum from venous blood, which is measured in most clinical laboratories.

In addition to the already mentioned sources of error, DEXTROSTIX will usually give somewhat erroneous readings below 50 mg/dl and above 250 mg/dl. These errors should not disturb the patient, because once control of BG is established, readings outside the 50–250 mg/dl range will rarely be encountered.

The details covered in this chapter may seem overwhelming, but so would the steps in driving a car if they were listed all at once. Yet, like operating a motor vehicle, BG measurement becomes automatic after a little practice. Measuring BG 6–8 times each day may also appear very time-consuming. In reality, the entire procedure should require less than two minutes for each BG, using DEXTRO-STIX, and less than three minutes per measurement with CHEMSTRIP bG. Thus the performance of 6–8 determinations usually involves perhaps 20 minutes per day, at most. Some patients have found that this is more than offset by the time recovered from reduction in sleep requirements when their BG is normalized.

10

THE GLUCOGRAF® DATA SHEET

SUMMARY

Essential to maintenance of normal BG is proper record keeping. The GLUCOGRAF Data Sheet was designed to display graphically all BG values measured in a week. If used according to the instructions given in this chapter, it will also permit patient or physician to identify readily the causes of any abnormal BG values so that preventive measures can be taken in the future. The reverse side of the Data Sheet contains a Meal Composition Record which may be of value during the first few weeks on our regimen. Both forms (Figs. 16 and 17) are printed in a full 8½-by-11-inch format suitable for photocopying.[1] These appear on pages 100–101 and 108–109.

The determination of BG perhaps 6–9 times each day is obviously not an end in itself. The resulting data is of little value unless recorded, analyzed, and acted upon. Although one purpose of BG monitoring is the immediate correction of deviations from ideal BG, there are two additional purposes:

1. Establishment of an initial insulin and diet regimen.
2. Continuous revision of the regimen as changes in life

---

1. Alternately, a pad containing one year's supply of GLUCOGRAF Data Sheets, punched with 3 holes for a loose-leaf binder, may be purchased from Sugar Free Center for Diabetics, 5623 Matilija Avenue, Van Nuys, Calif. 91401. The anticipated price is $7.50, including postage, for one pad, with substantial discounts for large orders.

style, stress, physiology, and other conditions may dictate. These changes may be very infrequent or may occur monthly as, for example, a result of the female menstrual cycle. There is no predicting when some changes in regimen may be required.

In order to achieve the desired purposes, a continuous record of pertinent data, together with a graph of BG values, is necessary. Therefore every patient should carry a GLU-COGRAF Data Sheet on his person (Figs. 15 and 16). On this sheet, the patient records not only all BG measurements, but also any information that will cast light on the causes for deviations from ideal BG.

Although some may question the need for data to be plotted on a graph, both patients and physicians have found it very convenient for spotting repeating BG abnormalities that might otherwise be lost in a maze of data. The GLU-COGRAF Data Sheet has been used by patients and physicians for more than a year and has been redesigned a number of times to yield the current version, which seems to meet the needs of many individuals.

One data sheet covers a patient's history for one week. It may be folded to one-eighth its size and carried in a pocket. After a week of data has been entered, the sheet may be stored folded in a standard 8½-by-5½-inch loose-leaf binder. If the patient wishes to use such a binder, he should secure an adjustable 3-hole punch for perforating the photocopies.

Figure 15 illustrates a GLUCOGRAF Data Sheet that has been partially filled out for a hypothetical patient. The following sections of this chapter serve to illustrate its proper use.

Abbreviations of Insulin Types

Because the Data Sheet allows very little space for entries, the insulin entries are abbreviated according to the following codes:

L   Lente insulin   R   Regular insulin
N   NPH insulin   S   Semilente insulin
P   Protamine Zinc insulin   UL   Ultralente insulin

A dose of 4 units Regular insulin mixed in the same syringe with 5 units Ultralente is recorded as 4R + 5UL. By entering the 4R before the 5UL we are indicating that the hypodermic syringe was *first* filled with 4 units of Regular insulin to which 5 units of Ultralente were subsequently added. It is important to indicate the sequence of filling when using a mixture. Up to 1 unit more than planned of the second insulin than the first insulin can actually be injected due to the "dead space" in the needle, if a permanently attached needle

DATA SHEET

GlucograF®

NAME	SUN.	MON.	TUES.

DATE WEEK BEGINS

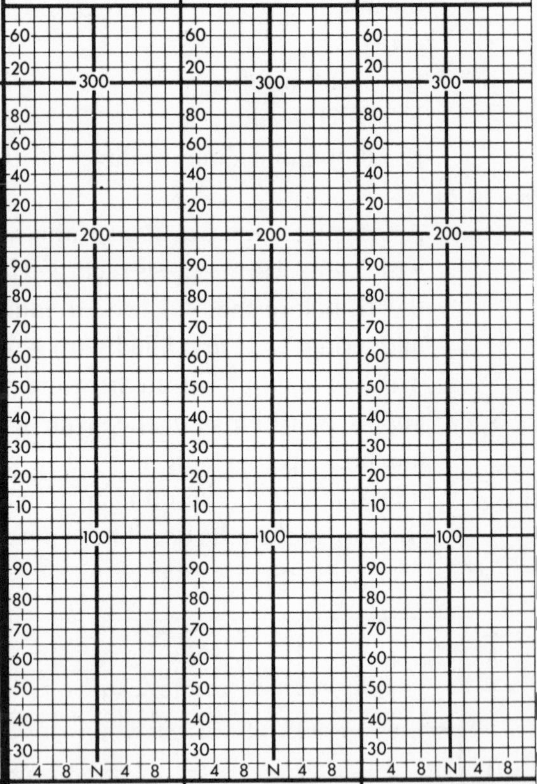

60
20
300
80
60
40
20
200
90
80
70
60
50
40
30
20
10
100
90
80
70
60
50
40
30
4 8 N 4 8

TIME—EVENT | TIME—EVENT | TIME—EVENT

DATA TO REMEMBER

1 Unit R will lower BG:_________mg/dl

USUAL INSULIN DOSES
Breakfast:

Lunch:

Supper:

BG EFFECTS OF SWEETS (mg/dl)

EXERCISE ADJUSTMENTS

WEIGHT PLAN

OTHER

©1981 R. Bernstein

WED.	THURS.	FRI.	SAT.

-60-	60-	60-	60-
-20-	20-	20-	20-
—300—	—300—	—300—	—300—
-80-	80-	80-	80-
-60-	60-	60-	60-
-40-	40-	40-	40-
-20-	20-	20-	20-
—200—	—200—	—200—	—200—
-90-	90-	90-	90-
-80-	80-	80-	80-
-70-	70-	70-	70-
-60-	60-	60-	60-
-50-	50-	50-	50-
-40-	40-	40-	40-
-30-	30-	30-	30-
-20-	20-	20-	20-
-10-	10-	10-	10-
—100—	—100—	—100—	—100—
-90-	90-	90-	90-
-80-	80-	80-	80-
-70-	70-	70-	70-
-60-	60-	60-	60-
-50-	50-	50-	50-
-40-	40-	40-	40-
-30-	30-	30-	30-

4 8 N 4 8	4 8 N 4 8	4 8 N 4 8	4 8 N 4 8
TIME—EVENT	TIME—EVENT	TIME—EVENT	TIME—EVENT

is used. Some removable needles may have such a large "dead space" that the dose difference can be up to 4 units. For consistent dosage when mixing insulins together in one syringe one must therefore stick to one type of needle/syringe combination and must always draw in the same insulin first.

When a usual dose of insulin is to be temporarily increased or decreased for some special reason, this is indicated by the use of parentheses as in the following examples:

(5 + 1)R + 7UL   Means that the usual dose of 5 units Regular insulin mixed with 7 units Ultralente has been supplemented by an extra unit of Regular.

(5−1)R + 7UL   Means that the usual dose has been reduced by 1 unit of Regular insulin so that only 4 units of Regular were administered with the usual 7 units of Ultralente.

"Data to Remember"

On the left-hand side of the form is a field surrounded by a dark border, headed DATA TO REMEMBER. This field will contain information that the patient may need during the course of the week. Since certain of these data (such as usual insulin doses) may change occasionally, the change may be too readily forgotten, especially if three different doses and two different insulins are being administered each day. Thus this special field is provided to substitute for memory. The following instructions pertain to sections of this field:

1. 1 Unit R Will Lower BG: _30_   mg/dl

All patients using the GLUCOGRAF method determine experimentally (see Chapter 12) the BG lowering effect of 1 unit of Regular insulin. For most adults with Type Ia (negligible C-peptide) diabetes, this will be about 30 mg/dl. Therefore this number has been entered above and on Fig. 15.

2. USUAL INSULIN DOSES

Breakfast: ~~6R+5UL~~
            Wed. ~~5½R+5UL~~
            Fri. 5R+5UL

Lunch: 4R

Supper: 6R+5UL

This section needs little explanation except to point out that the usual insulin dose may be changed during the week. Such a situation is shown here and in Fig. 15 for breakfast dose. The week began with a pre-breakfast dose of 6R + 5UL. On Wednesday it was reduced to 5½R + 5UL, and it was further reduced on Friday to 5R + 5UL. The first two doses were therefore crossed out but, for the sake of the record, not obliterated.

3. BG EFFECTS OF SWEETS (mg/dl) 1 Lifesaver = 10 mg/dl
                                  1 Dextrosol = 15
                                  1 Cherry = 4

Here is entered the calibrated BG increase (see Chapter 14) produced by the favorite candy, glucose tablet, or fruit for the treatment of hypoglycemia or for use while exercising. As explained later, fruits work too slowly for the proper treatment of hypoglycemia but may be fine for preventing hypoglycemia during exercise.

4. EXERCISE ADJUSTMENTS Biking = 1 Lifesaver every 2 miles.

This section serves as a reminder of what must be done to keep BG normal while exercising (see Chapter 15). The entries in this section will vary from patient to patient and from exercise to exercise. A football player may find that half an apple (fairly slow-acting) at the beginning of each quarter keeps his BG normal, while a marathon runner may require a glucose tablet (very fast-acting) every 10 minutes.

5. WEIGHT PLAN

Our regimen uses the weight of the patient as a guide to

changes in diet and insulin dose (see pages 160–163). This
section of the sheet is used to store any guidelines that the
healthcare provider may propose for weight maintenance or
control, such as ideal body weight, target weight, number of
pounds to be lost or gained per week, etc.

6. OTHER   *1 R for 3 slices Swiss cheese*

Bk fst: Hip
Lunch: Arm
Supper: Abdomen
Other times: Arm

This section is for any other information that the patient
may want to remember. In the example shown, the patient
likes to snack occasionally on Swiss cheese. He must, however, take 1 unit of R for every 3 slices, to prevent BG elevation when snacking.

This patient also observes that his insulin begins to act
more rapidly when injected in certain sites. He therefore, in
order to maintain a predictability of insulin action, reserves
certain injection sites for certain times of the day. He uses
this section of his chart to keep track of where he is to inject.

BG Graph

This field on the data sheet (Figs. 15, 16) is broken down
into 7 vertical columns, corresponding to the days of the
week. Every BG measurement is to be entered as a point on
this graph. At the end of each day the points for the day are
connected by straight lines—as shown in the Figures. The
numbers at the bottom of each column correspond to hours
of the day. Thus 4–8–N–4–8 stand for 4 A.M.–8 A.M.–12
noon–4 P.M.–8 P.M. Every small box in the left-to-right direction represents 2 hours. The long, vertical lines occur at
12 midnight and the short, heavy vertical lines occur at 12
noon. One o'clock in the morning, for example, would be in
the middle of the first box.

The vertically spaced numbers are BG values. The graph

covers BG from 20 mg/dl to 400 mg/dl. Below 200 mg/dl, every small box is 5 mg/dl. Between 200 and 300 mg/dl, every box is 10 mg/dl. Between 300 and 400 mg/dl, every box is 20 mg/dl.

Time-Event

At the bottom of each day's graph is a section headed TIME-EVENT. This is for the entry of every significant event that might affect BG, together with the time of the event. The following suggests the kinds of events that should be listed in these spaces:

1. Every BG measurement (and urine glucose measurements, until they are discontinued).

2. Every scheduled meal or snack. If the content of the meal or snack corresponds to the prescribed diet, no further notation is necessary. Any additions to or deletions from a meal or snack should be specifically indicated.

3. Every exercise session, including the starting and finishing times and the nature of exercise (for example, "1:30–2:00 Swim"). Patients engaged in cardio-respiratory development programs should also record their maximum heart rate (see pages 180–181) and the time period over which it was sustained.

4. Any unusual situations that might affect BG control, such as: "Virus—didn't eat all day," "Spent entire morning in airplane," "Extra meat at dinner," and so forth.

Following are examples of event entries, by a hypothetical patient, covering a 24-hour period, with explanations of these entries and brief comments in the right-hand column. Note how the patient uses arrows to indicate cause and effect or reasons for changes in insulin dose.

Entries		Translations
TIME-EVENT		
12:15 BG 120	½R	Just before bed BG was slightly elevated at 120 mg/dl, so patient injected ½ unit of

Entries	Translations
TIME-EVENT	
	Regular insulin to lower BG toward his target value of 100 mg/dl.
7:05 BG 105 6R + 5UL	When patient awoke BG was 105, so he administered his usual insulin dose of 6 units Regular mixed with 5 units Ultralente.
8:00 Bkfst.	55 minutes after taking insulin, patient ate his usual breakfast. He then biked 6 miles during which he consumed 3 LIFESAVER candies as
8:30 biked 6 mi., 3 LS	protection against hypoglycemia. Post-exercise BG was lower than his target value of 100 mg/dl, so patient ate 2 more LIFESAVERS to raise it. Note how he uses an
9:10 BG 80, 2 LS	arrow to indicate likely cause of low BG.
11:10 BG 98	Preprandial BG was near target value.
12:10 (5 + 1)R Will eat lunch out	The usual pre-lunch dose of 5 units Regular was increased by 1 unit because patient planned to eat at a restaurant and expected to consume more protein than in his usual lunch.
12:40 Lunch	Lunch *began* at 12:40.
4:15 BG 115	About 3 hours after finishing lunch, BG was measured to see how it was affected by meal. BG was only slightly above target, so no action was taken.
5:30 BG 118 ½R	1½ hours pre-dinner BG was still slightly above target. Patient therefore injected ½ unit Regular insulin.
6:00 Wgt. 145 lbs.	Patient weighed himself.
6:15 6R + 5UL	50 minutes before dinner, patient injected his usual pre-dinner dose of 6R + 5UL.
7:05 Dinner	Dinner *began* at 7:05.
10:00 BG 115 ½R 10:30 bed	BG at 10 P.M. served requirement to measure both BG at bedtime and 2–3 hours postprandially. Patient did not want the slight BG elevation to remain all night, so he took ½ unit of Regular insulin before bed.

We see, from the preceding example, that a well-kept Data Sheet is not just a history, but an active guide to what cause brings about what BG effect. Once a suitable insulin/ diet regimen has been worked out, neither patient nor physician need be perplexed about cause and effect, provided appropriate data is recorded. If the data exceed the available space in a TIME-EVENT column, continue on the reverse side where additional columns appear.

Meal Composition Record

Some physicians want certain patients to record everything they eat during the first few weeks of the GLU-COGRAF regimen. We therefore have provided the Meal Composition Record (Fig. 17). This form is also reproduced full size for photocopying on pages 108–109. If possible, the two forms should be reproduced on opposite sides of the same sheet. Patients who are no longer required to maintain meal records sometimes like to use the reverse side of the Data Sheet for shopping lists and other reminders.

GlucograF®

MEAL COMPOSITION RECORD			
NAME			
DATE WEEK BEGINS			
	SUN.	MON.	TUES.

© 1981
R. Bernstein

WED.	THURS.	FRI.	SAT.

11

TYPES OF INSULIN

SUMMARY

There are several ways of classifying the numerous insulins available in the U.S. and abroad:

1. Timing of BG lowering effect (Regular, Lente, NPH, Protamine Zinc, Ultralente, etc.).
2. Animal source (pork, beef, mixed pork and beef, synthetic human).
3. Strength or concentration (U-100, U-40, U-80, U-500, etc.).
4. Purity (single peak, single component).

Each of these classifications is considered in this chapter. Emphasis is on the timing of BG lowering effect, because comprehension of this characteristic is essential for a clear understanding of the insulin regimen presented in Chapter 12.

Timing of BG Lowering Effect

Insulins may be assigned to one of the following three categories, depending upon how rapidly or slowly they act on BG:

1. Rapid action.
2. Intermediate action.
3. Prolonged action.

The various insulins consist of the purified hormone treated with modifying substances to form tiny (microscopic) particles. The solubility of the insulin in tissue fluids and membranes depends upon the structure and size of these particles, which, in turn, depend upon the nature of the modifying ingredient. Those particles which are more soluble will permit insulin to make its way more rapidly into the blood. We thus have rapid-acting, prolonged-acting, and intermediate-acting insulins, depending upon the nature and amount of modifying substance. The insulins commonly used in the U.S. are listed in the table on page 112.

The timing of action shown for the various insulins is only approximate and will vary from patient to patient. For a given individual, timing will depend upon many factors, including:

1. Site of injection (thigh, arm, abdomen, hip) and how often that site receives insulin injections.

2. Amount injected.

3. Exercise of muscle underlying injection site.

4. Depth of injection (Regular insulin works faster if injected deeply).

5. BG level at time of injection, and simultaneous effect upon BG of meals, activity, and other insulins.

Several important observations should be made at this point:

1. The effect of any insulin on BG usually diminishes as BG rises. We call this the "nonlinear" response of BG to insulin. The BG level at which insulin begins to lose its full effect will vary from patient to patient.

2. A small portion of the injected insulin will become bound to proteins (mostly albumin) in the blood or tissues, which temporarily prevent it from acting. It usually is not released until many hours after the major portion has acted

MAJOR CHARACTERISTICS OF INSULINS AVAILABLE IN THE U.S.

Insulin Action	Generic American[1] Designation	Our Abbreviation	Appearance	Time BG Is Usually Affected (hours after injection)[2]			If Mixed in Same Syringe with Regular Insulin, the Regular Insulin Will Act Independently	Modified with Foreign Proteins
				Onset of Action	Maximum Action	Action Terminates		
Rapid	Regular	R	Clear	½–1½	2–3	4–7		No
	Semilente	S	Cloudy	1–2	3–5	6–9	Not tested.	No
	Lente	L	Cloudy	2–4	7–11	14–16	Provided ratio of R to L is greater than 3:1.	No
Intermediate	NPH	N	Cloudy	2–3	6–10	12–14	Provided ratio of R to N is equal to or greater than 1:1.	Yes
	Mixtard premixed 1:2 mixture of R and N		Cloudy	1½	4–9	12–14		Yes
Prolonged	Ultralente	UL	Cloudy	5–8	20–28	36–96	Yes—Mix at time of use. Do not premix.	No
	Protamine Zinc	P	Cloudy	6–8	16–22	24–72	No[3]	Yes

1. Foreign equivalents of insulins supplied in the U.S. are given in Appendix H.

2. Timing will vary from patient to patient, and with the site of injection and volume injected. The times shown can thus only be approximate.

3. Effects of mixing R and P range from virtually nil, when R:P ratio is less than 1:4, to creation of equivalent of NPH when ratio is 2:1.

on BG. The small portion so affected will vary considerably from patient to patient but typically may be about one-fifth of the injected dose. The timing of release of this protein-bound insulin is difficult to predict.

3. If an injection site is used very frequently, or if it contains scar tissue instead of fat, insulin may take longer to reach the bloodstream.

4. If muscle underlying an injection site is exercised vigorously, the rate of insulin absorption can be tripled.

5. The onset of action, for Regular insulin, appears to occur earlier at larger doses than at smaller ones. Furthermore, the magnitude of the peak will of course be greater at larger doses. Longer-acting insulins, unlike Regular, tend to begin acting earlier at lower doses.

6. Insulin absorption is slowed if the injection site is cold (for example, if patient stands outdoors in cold weather) and accelerated if the injection site is warm (for example, after a hot bath). This is due to the fact that local blood circulation is impaired by cold and enhanced by heat.

These six effects can be very significant and should be memorized by the patient.

The typical patient on our regimen will eventually be using both rapid-acting (Regular) and prolonged- or intermediate-acting insulins. In order to minimize the number of daily injections, two insulins are usually mixed together in the same syringe. When Regular insulin (R) is mixed with Ultralente (UL), the two act almost (but not quite) independently, as if they were injected separately. R and UL can be mixed immediately before use. If they are mixed hours or days prior to use, the insulin can lose some of its activity. When R is mixed with NPH insulin (N), the two will act more or less independently provided the dose of R equals or exceeds that of N. When R is added, in small proportions, to Protamine Zinc insulin (P), the resulting mixture has virtually the same timing as the original P.[1] In most cases, this mixture will serve no useful purpose, so R and P are mixed only for very special situations. If R is mixed with Lente (L) in ratios less than 3 parts R to 1 part L, the mixture can have a net action somewhere between those of L and R and the timing of action for any given ratio will be difficult to predict. Therefore we prefer N to L for mixing with R.

Two of the insulins—N and P—contain a modifier, called protamine, derived from fish sperm. Protamine effectively slows the action of Regular insulin. It is a "foreign" protein, differing considerably from any similar human protein, and can therefore cause allergic reactions in some patients. These reactions can vary from slight swelling or inflammation at the injection site to failure of BG to respond to the insulin. The latter occurrences are relatively rare.

Animal Source of the Insulin

Commercially prepared insulin is obtained from beef and/ or pork pancreatic tissue. Beef, pork, and human insulin all have similar but not identical molecular structures and each is composed of 51 amino acid building blocks connected together in a precise sequence. The sequence of amino acids in pork insulin is the same as that in human insulin, except that, at position 30, human insulin has the amino acid threonine, and pork insulin has the amino acid alanine. The sequence of amino acids in beef insulin, however, differs from that of human insulin at three positions. The expected effect of these differences would be that, in humans, pork insulin will frequently be more effective than beef insulin. Other anticipated effects relate to the possibility that these animal insulins may be treated as "foreign" proteins by the same

---

1. This is supposedly not true of neutral P made in Scandinavian countries. Mixtures of R and neutral P may behave almost as if the two insulins were injected separately.

human immune systems that attack invading viruses, bacterial toxins, and the like. Since beef insulin is more "foreign" than pork insulin, it is more likely to be inactivated. In reality, both beef and pork insulins cause at least a very small immune response in most humans. As expected, the partial inactivation of pork insulin by human immune mechanisms is far less frequent or intense than the inactivation of beef insulin. Nevertheless, a few individuals respond more favorably to beef insulin than to pork insulin.

Unless a vial of insulin is marked "BEEF" or "PORK" in large red letters, it will be a *mixture* of beef and pork insulins. In the U.S., pure beef or pure pork insulins are dispensed by pharmacies, upon special request and at somewhat greater cost.[2] Since many patients (perhaps 20 percent) will require considerably lower doses of pure pork or pure beef insulin, the demand for these special insulins (particularly pork) is growing rapidly. After switching from beef/pork insulin to either pure pork or pure beef, some patients experience a period of unpredictable BG swings that can last up to several months. During this period, it is wise to monitor BG even more frequently than is recommended in Chapter 9.

Ultralente insulin, the favored prolonged-action insulin for most patients on our regimen, is, due to the low demand until now, not made from pork insulin. Some patients who experience problems with the commercial beef/pork mixture are using instead pork Protamine Zinc insulin and separate injections of R.

Although not yet available in the marketplace, synthetic insulin having the same molecular structure as human insulin is now being tested on humans. If the current testing program is successful, this synthetic human insulin may be sold commercially within the next few years. Such insulin will be

---

2. Recently two European manufacturers, Nordisk and Novo, began to distribute their insulins in the U.S.A. All Nordisk insulins and three Novo insulins—Actrapid®, Semitard®, and Monotard®—are pure pork formulations.

of value principally to patients who show an allergic response to animal insulins or to some patients who require unduly large doses of animal insulins. It is also possible that the phenomenon of temporary antibody binding of insulin (see item 2, pages 111 and 113) may not occur in many patients who use the new insulin.

Strength or Concentration of Insulin

Strength of insulin is specified in "units per cubic centimeter (cc)." Outside the U.S., up to four different strengths or concentrations of insulins are commercially available. In the U.S., only three of the four following concentrations can be obtained:

1. *Highest concentration:* "U-500," 500 units per cc, is available in the U.S., on special order only, in Regular pork insulin and may be used by patients requiring very high doses. This strength tends to often have a prolonged activity resembling that of Lente or NPH insulins.

2. *Most commonly used concentration in U.S.:* "U-100," 100 units per cc.

3. *Most commonly used concentration outside the U.S.:* "U-80," 80 units per cc, no longer available in the U.S.

4. *Low dose concentration:* "U-40," 40 units per cc. Some patients, such as infants and those who still produce considerable amounts of endogenous insulin, will show very large BG reductions (perhaps 60–100 mg/dl), after injection of only 1 unit of insulin. These patients cannot tolerate even a ½-unit error in the measurement of their very small insulin dose. One solution to this problem is a low-strength insulin, such as U-40. There is a possibility that in the U.S., the FDA may decertify this concentration on the grounds that three concentrations of insulin (U-40, U-100, and U-500) on the market might confuse patients and lead to erroneous dosage

measurement. This can occur, for example, if U-40 insulin is administered from a U-100 insulin syringe.

Disposable Insulin Syringes

Disposable hypodermic insulin syringes are available in the U.S. for use with U-100 and U-40 insulins only. Syringes for U-40, U-80, and U-100 insulins are available outside the U.S. A given insulin strength should be used only with the corresponding syringe—except that U-500 insulin may be used in a U-100 syringe, provided that all numbers on the syringe are multiplied by 5.

Recently ½-cc disposable U-100 insulin syringes, that are almost as long as, but narrower than, the older 1-cc syringes, have become available. The syringe has a printed scale with markings for every unit. Intermediate doses, such as 2½ units, can be estimated with good accuracy. These new syringes used with U-100 insulin comprise the combination recommended for most patients on our regimen, for the reason that accuracy of measurement is combined with small volumes of injected insulin. Smaller injections are not only less painful but the sites heal more rapidly, and the injections are less likely to cause damage to fatty, subcutaneous tissue, thus tending to act on BG with greater predictability of timing.

In the extreme case of a patient requiring less than 5 units per day of injected insulin, the pharmacist can prepare U-50 insulin by adding U-100 insulin to a sterile vial containing an equal volume of diluting fluid.[3] This mixture can be administered with a ½-cc U-100 syringe if every marking is read as ½ unit instead of 1 unit. The use of specially prepared U-50 insulin doubles the accuracy with which very small doses can be measured. The accuracy will be greater than that attained by using U-40 insulin in a 1-cc U-40 syringe. (Half-cc disposable syringes are not available for U-40 insulin.) A pharma-

---

3. Diluting fluid and sterile mixing vials are available from Eli Lilly & Co.

cist can also prepare U-25 and U-10 insulins for use in very rare cases such as diabetic infants.

Purity of Insulin

Commercially prepared insulins may contain a small percentage of proinsulin, glucagon, and other non-insulin substances. Most insulin made in the U.S. comes in a high-purity solution, called *single peak* insulin, that contains less than 1 percent of these impurities. Some patients who display allergic response to even single-peak pork insulin may do better with a higher-purity solution called *single component* pork insulin. This insulin has minuscule amounts of impurities and is made in the U.S. as ILETIN II, pork (Lilly; also available in pure beef insulins). The Novo and Nordisk pork insulins distributed in the U.S. and abroad are all of "single component" purity. Single-component beef insulin may be ordered by physicians on an experimental basis (at no charge). Single-component insulins are standard in many countries outside the U.S.

Insulin Lipodystrophies

Insulin is usually injected into subcutaneous (under the skin) fat pads. Frequent injection into the same site can cause unattractive depressions in the skin surface, called lipoatrophy (loss of fat) or equally disfiguring lumps, called lipohypertrophy (enlargement of fat cells). These "lipodystrophies" may not disappear unless the affected site is not injected for a number of years. An alternative treatment has been to substitute the high-purity single-component insulins for the insulins formerly used. Lipoatrophy can actually be reversed by repeatedly injecting single-component insulins into the skin depressions, until they fill in. Lipodystrophies are more

common in children, adolescent girls, and in patients injecting large doses of insulin.

Insulin dosage can sometimes be reduced and lipodystrophies prevented, by the use of single-component pork insulin
and by using the insulin and dietary regimens described in
Chapters 12 and 13. These regimens will both lower the total
daily insulin dose and greatly reduce the volume injected at
one time, because the daily dose will be divided into three
injections. The sites of these small injections heal very rapidly, and usually cannot be located several hours after injection, even by the patient.

12

THE PHYSIOLOGIC USE OF INSULIN

SUMMARY

A major factor in maintaining normal BG is the use of insulin in amounts and with a timing that mimics the B-cell insulin response of the nondiabetic. Optimum initial success has been achieved in most Type Ia diabetics with the following trial dosage schedule:

Before breakfast: (Body weight in kg) × (1/10R + 1/10 UL)
Before lunch: (Body weight in kg) × (1/10R)
Before supper: (Body weight in kg) × (1/10R + 1/10 UL)

Suggestions are given in this chapter for adapting this basic schedule to individual needs and to insulins other than UL. The recommended insulin regimens will function properly only in conjunction with the low-carbohydrate/high-protein diet described in Chapter 13. It is also necessary that R be given whenever BG is found to be elevated.

The topics covered in this chapter include:

1. The nonlinear response of BG to insulin.
2. The basic insulin regimen.
3. Calibrating action time of Regular insulin.
4. The patient who responds too rapidly to preprandial Regular insulin.
5. Approaches to initiating the basic insulin regimen.
6. Special situations that may require other insulins instead of Ultralente.

7. Working with NPH or Lente when their action is too brief.

8. Eliminating the 16–22 hour peak when using Protamine Zinc insulin.

9. The use of Regular insulin in calibrated amounts to correct blood glucose elevation.

10. Accelerating the action of Regular insulin.

11. The cumulative effect of injected insulin.

12. Two more possible benefits of physiologic insulin dosage.

13. Trading units for minutes.

14. Insulin usage and the individual patient.

The physiologic use of insulin is merely an attempt to mimic, with exogenous (injected) insulin, the performance of the normal pancreatic B-cell in its efforts to control BG. This implies the use of very small doses, timed in such a manner that BG remains almost continually within the normal range.

Injected insulin does not enter the bloodstream immediately, unless it is injected into a vein, yet certain foods (carbohydrates) can cause BG to rise within minutes after they are consumed. It is therefore necessary to time insulin administration in anticipation of eating. It is also necessary to adhere to a diet that will not produce a more rapid postprandial BG rise than can be controlled by injected insulin. Dietary considerations are covered in Chapter 13. The concurrent use of insulin to achieve the goal of continually normal BG is considered in this chapter.

Throughout the remainder of this book, the normal BG range will be assumed as 80–120 mg/dl. In reality, nondiabetics can frequently experience BG levels both below and above this range. Our normal range was chosen to be narrower than that of the general population because many individuals whose BG is in the normal range begin to experience uncomfortable hypoglycemic symptoms at 75 mg/dl, while some find that once BG exceeds 130 mg/dl, it may begin to drift upward, as explained in the following section.

The Nonlinear Response of BG to Insulin

At higher BG levels, insulin becomes less effective in its capacity to lower BG. For example, at a BG of 130 mg/dl, 1 unit of Regular insulin might lower BG by 30 mg/dl. For the same patient, at a BG of 400 mg/dl, 1 unit of Regular insulin might lower BG by only 15 mg/dl. The reasons for this "nonlinear" response of BG to insulin are not known for certain but are believed to be related to high blood levels of counter-regulatory hormones such as glucagon and glucocorticoids. Secretion of certain counter-regulatory hormones is inhibited by insulin. When BG is elevated, there is usually inadequate insulin present, and blood levels of counter-regulatory hormones are free to rise. Once these levels are high, the insulin required for a given BG drop will increase. Without extra insulin BG will continue to rise. Thus a high BG will be followed by a higher BG, unless adequate insulin is administered.

If the preceding reasoning is correct, we can draw at least two additional important conclusions:

1. If no insulin is present, BG will rise (due to counter-regulation), even if BG was initially normal and patient is fasting.

2. If a patient has taken a dose of insulin that will usually maintain a normal BG, this dose will not be adequate to prevent an elevated BG from rising still further. Thus more insulin would be required to maintain a constant BG of 200 mg/dl, than to maintain a constant BG of 100 mg/dl. This is one of the reasons why so many diabetics require more insulin than the nondiabetic produces. If BG is maintained in the "normal" range, insulin requirements will be lower and BG will also be easier to control.

In practice, these two conclusions turn out to be not only valid, but extremely important. To achieve success at BG control, the patient must appreciate their significance, as they are the underlying reasons for our unusual regimen.

The Basic Insulin Regimen

Let us now further consider BG regulation in the non-diabetic, together with our scheme for using injected insulin to mimic this regulation for the diabetic.

If a nondiabetic fasts for 24 hours and does not engage in strenuous exercise, his B-cells will continually produce a nearly steady but minute flow of insulin granules. In the course of a day, roughly 2/10 unit of insulin will be produced for every kilogram (2.2 pounds) of body weight (1/10 unit per pound) in the typical nonobese, nondiabetic, fasting adult. We can duplicate this in the fasting, totally insulin-dependent (Type Ia, Chapter 6), non-insulin-resistant, non-pregnant, nonobese adult diabetic, by injecting a daily dose of *2/10 unit Ultralente insulin (UL) per kg* (1/10 unit/lb) of body weight. We choose UL rather than the other prolonged- or intermediate-acting insulins because it has the most uniform action over time, with but a very shallow peak (see table, page 112). If injected in *2 half-doses per day*, spaced approximately 12 hours apart, UL will provide a steady, continuous release of insulin to the bloodstream—just as the healthy B-cell does. Thus if a patient weighs 65 kg (143 pounds), his daily dose of UL might be 65 × 2/10 = 13 units.[1] It would probably be administered in two injections of 6½ units each. To minimize the injected volume of liquid while still maintaining an accurate measurement of dose, we would use U-100 insulin (because it's more concentrated than U-40) and a ½-cc U-100 disposable syringe (because it has a scale that can be read more accurately than that of the

---

1. A person who exercises strenuously and regularly might require about 25 percent less UL.

more commonly used 1-cc syringe) (see Chapter 11, page 117). It is important to note, when adjusting dosage of UL, that changes in the A.M. dose may not affect BG until the night, and changes in the P.M. dose may not affect BG until the following morning or afternoon. The actual timing will be different for different patients.

The typical day for diabetics and nondiabetics is, of course, not one of fasting. It can be viewed, however, as a fast interrupted by meals. As the digestion of a meal proceeds in a nondiabetic, the normal B-cell will produce a substantial release of insulin granules. The net result in the nondiabetic is a slight postprandial BG rise, but still within a reasonably normal range—perhaps from 90 mg/dl preprandial to 125 mg/dl postprandial and then back to 90 mg/dl after 2–3 hours. In the totally insulin-dependent diabetic (Type Ia), the postprandial BG rise can be very great—perhaps several hundred mg/dl—clearly necessitating further measures in addition to the Ultralente. We can reduce this postprandial rise to virtually zero by a combination of Regular insulin injected at a planned time interval before a meal, and a diet that offers minimal glucose challenge (see Chapter 13).

In practice, the totally insulin-dependent, non-insulin-resistant, nonobese adult diabetic will require approximately *1/10 unit of R per kg of body weight* (1/20 unit per lb) *prior to every meal,* provided that the diet outlined in Chapter 9 is followed. R is used because it is the fastest-acting insulin available. In most cases, the R should be mixed in the same syringe with UL prior to breakfast and prior to the evening meal, so that both meals and between-meal fasts are covered by insulin. The R should be drawn into the syringe before the UL is added. Before the midday meal, only R should be injected.

Let us now set forth a typical daily insulin regimen per kilogram of body weight, based on the preceding guidelines.

We will use the abbreviations for insulin doses that were introduced in Chapter 10.

Before breakfast: 1/10R + 1/10UL per kg.
Before lunch: 1/10R   per kg.
Before supper: 1/10R + 1/10UL per kg.

Total dose: 3/10R + 2/10UL = 5/10 = ½ unit per kg per day.

This total dose of ½ unit per kg per day is roughly the insulin output of the nondiabetic, nonfasting adult pancreas over the same period of time. Let us now apply this dosage scheme to our "typical" nonexercising, non-insulin-resistant nonobese, Type Ia diabetic adult. We will multiply all of the doses by his body weight of 65 kg (143 lb).

Before breakfast: 65 × (1/10R + 1/10UL) = 6½R + 6½UL
Before lunch: 65 × (1/10R)   = 6½R
Before supper: 65 × (1/10R + 1/10UL) = 6½R + 6½UL

Total daily insulin: 19½ R + 13UL = 32½ units
                                                           per day

If the patient were exercising strenuously for one hour every day, we would lower only his UL by perhaps 25 percent of each dose regardless of the time of day at which he exercises (see Chapter 15). This would give a total daily dose of 19½R + 10UL = 29½ *units per day.* This is a rough approximation of the amount of insulin required by a nonobese, nonpregnant, non-insulin-resistant,[2] exercising, 65-kg diabetic who has absolutely no endogenous insulin production (zero C-peptide).

If a patient fits these specifications and is taking doses greater than 20 percent above the guidelines, the most likely cause is an inappropriate approach to diet and insulin. Insu-

---

2. Including transient insulin resistance caused by birth control pills or other drugs.

lin "resistance" is possible but occurs in very few cases. On the other hand, if insulin requirements are less than 80 percent of these guidelines, C-peptide levels should be checked, because this patient may still have functioning B-cells producing endogenous insulin.

Any meal may be skipped or reduced, provided the preprandial dose of R is also skipped or reduced. Meals need not follow a fixed schedule. UL doses should not be skipped.

Calibrating Action Time of Regular Insulin

Essential to our insulin regimen is proper timing of injection of R prior to meals. The R must begin to enter the bloodstream just as the glucose digested from the carbohydrate part of the meal enters the bloodstream. If this is planned properly, BG will remain approximately *unchanged* during and after the meal. If BG is outside the target range at any time after a meal, something is being done incorrectly. The length of time that a patient should wait for a meal after injecting R will vary with the individual. It can be determined experimentally, before a meal, as follows:

1. Measure BG. (If BG exceeds 200 mg/dl, experimental results will be altered by the "nonlinear" response to insulin and the experiment will not be valid.)

2. Wait 30 minutes and measure BG again, to make sure that BG is not drifting up or down.

3. If BG did not change, inject preprandial dose of R or of R + UL. This test should actually be performed once for R alone (lunch) and once for R + UL (supper) because the addition of UL may slow the onset of activity of the mixed R.

4. Wait 30 minutes, then measure BG again.

5. Continue measuring BG every 15 minutes, recording the time, until BG has dropped 10 mg/dl from the starting

value. The expired time after injection of R is the *maximum* appropriate preprandial waiting period. BG will drop rapidly if the meal is not started at this point.

Most patients have a preprandial waiting period of from 30 minutes to 75 minutes. The shorter wait usually applies to Type Ib or Type II patients who are producing some endogenous insulin, or to Type Ia patients who limit their carbohydrate intake to high-fiber vegetables totaling less than 1 bread exchange per meal (see Chapter 13). The 75-minute wait is more likely to apply to some Type Ia patients who are not only producing no insulin in response to meals but may also have certain forms of insulin resistance.

For a given patient, the six factors listed on pages 111 and 113 that affect rate of insulin absorption still apply and should be remembered. They can be of use creatively to deliberately speed up or slow down absorption of R to satisfy special timetables. For example, exercising or massaging the injection site might speed absorption considerably.

The Patient Who Responds Too Rapidly to Preprandial Regular Insulin

On rare occasions, a patient is encountered for whom blood levels of preprandial R develop very rapidly and dissipate very rapidly after injection. Such an individual first develops hypoglycemia and later, as protein is digested from the meal, develops hyperglycemia. The solution to this problem is to use preprandial Semilente instead of R. For this purpose, Semilente should not be mixed with UL or other insulins but should be injected separately.

Approaches to Initiating the Basic Insulin Regimen

In using Ultralente insulin, we must not forget that activity can continue for as long as 96 hours after injection.

When a patient is first introduced to UL, it might take about 3 days before the full cumulative effect on BG is secured. Therefore, it may be necessary to supplement the UL, during the first 2 days, with a number of additional small doses of R, depending upon BG measurements.

Considering this slow cumulative effect of UL, when making small adjustments in dosage, the patient should wait 3 days to observe the effect on BG before adjusting the dose further. If possible, changes in dose of either UL or R should be gradual and should not exceed 1–2 units per injection— except where the patient is either clearly insulin-resistant or grossly hypoglycemic. Dosage changes of ½ unit at a time are perfectly reasonable.

The "typical" values (per kg) of daily insulin requirements, cited earlier in this chapter, apply to many Type Ia patients and can be used as trial starting points for some patients. Remember, however, that basic long-acting insulin requirements can be reduced:

1. If there is some endogenous insulin production (C-peptide in urine or blood).
2. During certain phases of the menstrual cycle. The phases vary from one patient to another. For example, one patient may require more insulin on the day of ovulation and another may require less insulin that day.
3. Postpartum (after delivery of baby).
4. By weight-reduction diets.
5. During treatment with certain pharmaceuticals, including large doses of aspirin.
6. If patient exercises regularly at least several times per week.

Insulin requirements can be increased:

1. During growth spurts.
2. If patient is obese.

3. During certain phases of menstrual cycle.
4. During pregnancy.
5. By infection or illness.
6. By other immune and nonimmune causes of insulin resistance, including allergy to injected insulin, miscellaneous endocrine disorders, etc.
7. During treatment with certain drugs, including steroids and oral contraceptives.
8. During diets designed for weight gain.
9. During hospitalization or surgery.
10. By emotional or physiological stress.[3]
11. When BG is chronically elevated.

Because so many factors can affect the basic insulin dose and because we don't want to begin the new regimen with frequent hypoglycemia, it is proper to devise a new *trial* regimen according to whichever of the following methods yields the *lowest* total daily insulin dose.

Method I. 1/10 unit of UL mixed with 1/10 unit of R per kilogram (2.2 lb) of body weight, prior to breakfast and prior to evening meal. In addition, 1/10 unit of R per kilogram of body weight, prior to midday meal. Reduce all doses of UL by 25 percent if patient exercises regularly and strenuously.

Method II. Start with the total daily dose of all types of insulin prescribed for the patient under his old regimen. Reduce this total by one-third to get a new daily dose, which we here call "dose." This should then be administered as follows:

Before breakfast: 1/5 dose R mixed with 1/5 dose UL.
Before midday meal: 1/5 dose R.
Before evening meal: 1/5 dose R mixed with 1/5 dose UL.

---

3. It is uncommon for chronic emotional stress to *directly* cause a prolonged increase in insulin requirements of Type Ia patients. More frequently we see chronic stress leading to increased eating which creates a need for more insulin. On the other hand, severe emotional stress lasting but a few hours can readily lead to elevated BG.

Let's use the preceding guidelines to work out a trial insulin regimen for a hypothetical patient, Albert Ramsbottom. Mr. Ramsbottom weighs 70 kg, which is below his ideal body weight. He is currently taking two doses per day of NPH mixed with R such that all of his N and R added together totals 45 units of insulin per day. Mr. Ramsbottom is a lion tamer and spends several hours each day working with his lion—moderately strenuous exercise.

Method I (based on 70 kg body weight)

Before breakfast:	70 kg × (1/10R + 1/10UL) =	7R +	7UL
Before lunch:	70 kg × (1/10R) =	7R	
Before supper:	70 kg × (1/10R + 1/10UL) =	7R +	7UL
Uncorrected total	=	21R +	14UL
Less correction for exercise			
(25 percent × 14UL)		–	3UL
Corrected daily total		21R +	11UL = *32 units*

Method II (based on current insulin dose of 45 units per day less ⅓)
New "dose" = 45 (1 – ⅓) = 45 × ⅔ = 30 units per day

Before breakfast:	30 × (1/5R + 1/5UL)	=	6R + 6UL
Before lunch:	30 × (1/5R)	=	6R
Before supper:	30 × (1/5R + 1/5UL)	=	6R + 6UL
Daily total		18R +	12UL = *30 units*

Since Method I results in 32 units per day and Method II yields 30 units per day, Mr. Ramsbottom will follow the dosage schedule of Method II—the one that gave the lower total daily dose.

Special Situations That May Require Other Insulins Instead of Ultralente

Other insulins may produce more satisfactory results than UL for the following types of patients:

1. *Pregnant IDDM.* Insulin requirements may change very rapidly during pregnancy and immediately after delivery. UL continues acting for 1½–4 days after injection. It may therefore be wise to switch from UL to NPH or Lente,

both of which terminate their action in less than 1 day. NPH appears preferable to Lente because the independent action of R vanishes in mixtures with Lente unless there is at least 3 times as much R as Lente in the mixture.

2. *Patients who may be very active physically throughout the daytime hours* may require lower blood levels of insulin between meals during the day than at night. In such cases either of the following two approaches can be tried:

    a. Substitute NPH or possibly Lente for UL, reducing the pre-breakfast dose.

    b. Equally reduce both morning and evening doses of UL. Add Lente to the evening dose so that fasting blood levels of insulin at night will be greater than during the day.

3. *Patients who require much less insulin, when taking pure pork or pure beef insulin rather than the usual beef/pork mixture.* Since UL is currently unavailable in pure pork, NPH pork insulin or (if absolutely necessary) Lente or Protamine Zinc pork insulins may be substituted. Remember, however, that except in very special situations, neither L nor P should be mixed with R, which must be injected from a separate syringe. Thus a patient who uses L or P must take at least 5 daily injections: 2 before breakfast, 1 before lunch, and 2 before supper.

Working with NPH or Lente When Their Action Is Too Brief

As indicated in the preceding section, it may be desirable to try NPH or Lente insulins for certain patients. These intermediate-acting insulins when used for *both* daily doses may not yield adequate blood levels throughout the day in some patients. In perhaps half the cases we have seen, the action time of NPH (often less than 14 hours) is just too brief. This may also be true of Lente, which we rarely recommend. Remember that the timing of activity of any insulin can vary considerably from one patient to the next.

When NPH or Lente insulins are used instead of UL for *both* daily doses, the morning and evening doses must be spaced 11–13 hours (for some people, exactly 12 hours) apart to maintain the desired blood levels of insulin. This spacing may be inconvenient to some patients, because the two doses of NPH are mixed with R and the scheduling of R depends upon mealtime. Thus, when using NPH, we are obliging the patient to space breakfast and dinner about 12 hours apart. This inconvenience can be circumvented by administering the evening dose as 2 separate injections—R before the meal, and NPH or Lente 12 hours after the morning injection. Consider how this is done in the following example:

A patient arises daily at 7:30 A.M., administers a mixture of R + NPH insulins at 7:30 A.M., and starts breakfast at 8:30 A.M. He likes to dine at 5:30 P.M. and therefore must inject R at about 4:30 P.M., only 9 hours after his morning dose of NPH. If he were to add his evening NPH to the 4:30 dose of R, there would be a delay of 15 hours before his next morning dose of NPH. This would cause uneven blood insulin levels, resulting in possible hypoglycemia near midnight and elevated BG when awaking the following morning. The patient is therefore advised to take his evening NPH at 7:30 P.M., not to mix it with the R he takes at 4:30 P.M. Many patients will consider the extra injection less of an annoyance than rescheduling the evening meal. (Were Lente used instead of NPH, extra injections would probably be necessary anyway, because L and R do not mix with suitable timing in the dosage ratios that we are considering.)

If an intermediate-acting insulin maintains an effective blood level for less than 12 hours, as is the case for some patients, these patients have two choices (other than using UL):

1. Take the intermediate insulin in 3 doses (instead of 2) spaced exactly 8 hours apart. The pre-breakfast dose (if NPH) can be mixed with R (to save an extra injection) but the

other two doses are not likely to occur at lunchtime or sup-
pertime so R will have to be injected separately.

2. Use Protamine Zinc insulin (P) instead of an intermediate insulin. P should be administered at the same time and in
the same dose as UL. Pork P may require as little as a one-
third smaller dose than UL. Do not mix the preprandial doses
of R with the P but inject them from separate syringes.

Eliminating the 16–22 Hour Peak When Using Protamine Zinc Insulin

Protamine Zinc insulin will maintain blood insulin levels
in most patients for at least 24 hours. In many, however, it
has a peak of activity about 16–22 hours after injection. This
means that users are in danger of experiencing hypoglycemia
at night while sleeping, as a result of the P that was injected
in the morning. There are at least two ways of avoiding this
nocturnal hypoglycemia:

1. The classic method, dating back to the 1930s, is to eat a
protein snack (for example, 2 ounces of cheese) immediately
before retiring at night. The protein is very slowly converted
to glucose which opposes the hypoglycemia later on. This
technique works, but it is inconvenient to many patients—
especially those who are trying to lose weight.

2. An alternate solution to this problem is to flatten out
the peak of P activity by replacing about half the P with R.
The following example illustrates this technique:

Regimen with 16–22 Hour Peak	Eliminating 16–22 Hour Peak

Before breakfast: 5P, 5R
  (2 separate injections)
	(2½P + 2½R); 5R
	  (2 separate injections)

Before lunch: 5R	5R

Before supper: 5P, 5R
  (2 separate injections)
	(2½P + 2½R); 5R
	  (2 separate injections)

The use of equal amounts of P and R is not inflexible. Some people will require a bit more R with less P or vice versa. Just remember that a ratio of 1 part P to 2 parts R is the formula for NPH insulin.

Regular Insulin in Calibrated Amounts to Correct Blood Glucose Elevation

Even with a theoretically perfect combination of insulin and dietary regimens, unforeseen factors will continually cause slight, unpredicted variations in BG during the day. Such factors include unplanned changes in physical activity, poor estimation of food intake, site of insulin injection, and so on. In order to catch these BG variations before they become excessive, the patient must continue to perform multiple daily measurements of BG. As soon as BG reaches the extremes of our "normal" range (80–120 mg/dl), corrective action must be taken. Correction of *low* BG is covered in Chapter 14. Correction of *elevated* BG is discussed here.

First, however, we must reevaluate the normal range in terms of the patient's comfort. Many patients have had high BG levels for so long that they feel uncomfortable or hypoglycemic when BG drops below, possibly, 150 mg/dl. For such patients, a temporary "normal" range of 150–190 mg/dl may be desirable. This range can then be gradually reduced to 80–120 mg/dl over a period of 1–3 months. We shall, for convenience, base our recommendations on a "normal" range of 80–120 mg/dl with a target value of 100 mg/dl.[4]

If any BG measurement equals or exceeds 120 mg/dl, a small dose of R should be injected immediately, for the purpose of bringing BG to normal as rapidly as possible. If it is time for a preprandial dose anyway, the extra R can be added to this dose. If it is bedtime, the extra R should still be admin-

---

4. A small percentage of people do not feel hypoglycemic until BG drops to, say, 40 mg/dl, and feel "sick" when BG exceeds perhaps 110 mg/dl. Such patients will be more comfortable if their target BG is in the neighborhood of 80 mg/dl.

istered because the hazard of nocturnal hypoglycemia present under the old one- or two-dose regimens is no longer significant.

How is the proper amount of this extra dose of R determined? This is done by means of a simple experiment, designed to measure the effect on BG of 1 unit of R for Type Ia patients:

1. Select a convenient time and place, so that the experiment can proceed for about 4 hours without interruption. It should begin about 3 hours after a meal.

2. Measure BG. It should be above 120 mg/dl (to avoid hypoglycemia) and below 200 mg/dl (to avoid the nonlinear response of BG to insulin described at the beginning of this chapter).

3. Wait 30 minutes and measure BG again. It should be the same as the prior BG. If it has changed by more than 5 mg/dl, wait another 30 minutes and try again, or postpone the experiment.

4. Inject 1 unit of R if BG is 120–180 mg/dl. Inject 2 units of R if BG is 180–200 mg/dl.

5. Measure BG again after:

> 1½ hours
> 2 hours
> 3 hours
> 3½ hours
> 4 hours (if possible)

6. Using the last BG measurement of step 5, compute the amount that BG has dropped. Divide this by the number of units injected. The value obtained tells you how many mg/dl 1 unit of R will lower BG.

7. Repeat the experiment on several different days, to confirm the results.[5]

---

5. Patients using jet injectors to administer insulin may find that they cannot obtain consistent results from one day to the next. This may be due to the fact that some of the insulin administered with certain of these devices will leak out of the injection site in amounts that cannot be predicted. If results are inconsistent, switch to standard hypodermic syringes.

Type Ib or Type II patients should initially experiment with half the insulin doses indicated.

Estimating Calibration Without an Experiment

After a while, the physician can develop a knack for estimating the calibration of 1 unit of R, without requiring the preceding experiment. The following guidelines can be helpful in this respect:

1. For a 60-kg (132-lb) Type Ia (no C-peptide) nonpregnant, nonobese, non-insulin-resistant adult, 1 unit of R will usually lower BG by 30 mg/dl. The effect will be proportionately greater for lower body weight and less for greater body weight.

2. If a 60-kg patient is insulin-resistant (not merely overtreated with insulin), divide 900 mg/dl by the basic daily insulin dose (computed in the preceding section, and then approximated by trial and error). Example: An insulin-resistant patient requires 90 units as a basic daily dose (900 mg/dl ÷ 90 = 10 mg/dl). One unit of R will lower this patient's BG approximately 10 mg/dl.

3. If a 60-kg patient is producing endogenous insulin (C-peptide is present in substantial amounts) and therefore falls into Type Ib or Type II, proceed as in step 2. Example: A Type Ib patient requires 15 units as a basic daily dose (900 mg/dl ÷ 15 = 60 mg/dl). One unit of insulin will lower BG about 60 mg/dl.

4. Insulin effect is approximately proportional to the inverse of body weight. A patient weighing 75 kg would therefore expect 60/75 or about 4/5 the insulin effect of a similar patient weighing 50 kg.

5. If a patient requires less than 15 units per day, great care should be taken in using R, and serious consideration should be given to prescribing U-40 insulin or diluting fluid, as indicated on page 117. Either method will enable the patient to measure fractions of a unit easily.

As mentioned a number of times, insulin is usually less effective at higher BG levels. Therefore, 1 unit of R cannot be expected to have the same calibrated effect at a BG of 300 mg/dl that it has at 150 mg/dl. The approximate BG, where insulin effect begins to substantially deviate from the original calibration, may vary from patient to patient and from time to time. It appears, for many, to be in the 160–300 mg/dl range. The uncertainty of effect of insulin at elevated BG is yet another important reason for maintaining BG in the "normal" range.

The calibration for 1 unit of R should be entered in the space provided in the GLUCOGRAF form. If the calibration changes, the old one should be crossed out and the new one entered.

Accelerating the Action of Regular Insulin

Some patients may become impatient with the time delay between the injection of R and the lowering of an elevated BG. This delay can be especially annoying if BG is elevated prior to a meal, thus forcing an inconvenient postponement of eating.

Such delays can be shortened by a variety of techniques:

1. Vigorous prolonged massage of the site of subcutaneous injection will speed absorption.

2. Vigorous exercise of the muscle underlying the site of injection will also speed absorption.

3. Injecting R into a muscle (intramuscularly) can speed absorption by 30–50 percent over the subcutaneous route.

4. Injecting R into a vein (intravenously) can bring about very rapid BG response.

Intramuscular (IM) or intravenous (IV) injection should be undertaken only after thorough instruction by a clinician on the technique of administration. Both IM and IV injection may be more painful than the familiar subcutaneous (Sub Q) route of insulin administration. In people who are not obese these injections can be performed with the 27-gauge, ½-inch needle that comes with disposable insulin syringes. Obese individuals may require longer needles of the same gauge.

When injected IM or IV, a given dose of R will not only lower BG sooner but may lower it *more* than when injected Sub Q, because a considerable portion of Sub Q insulin is degraded at the injection site. For this reason it is imperative that initial calibration of the timing and BG effects of IM or IV injections be done in the presence of a health care professional. There is no sense in being exposed to the possibility of rapid-onset hypoglycemia without professional help in the immediate vicinity. A further mandatory precaution for the initial calibration is to use only half the dose of R than would have been used Sub Q for the same reduction of BG.

Even if the routine use of the IM route for the injection of R is not in the treatment plan for a patient, the IM injection and calibration of at least one dose (in the presence of a professional) can be of great value. It demonstrates to the patient the feel of an IM injection from a 27-gauge, ½-inch needle. Many patients occasionally inject insulin IM thinking that they are injecting it Sub Q. To someone with slim or average build, there may be very little difference in techniques between injecting IM or Sub Q. Yet the difference in absorption rate and amount can be so great as to be life-threatening—that is, cause rapid-onset, prolonged hypoglycemia.

Neither long-acting nor intermediate-acting insulins should be injected IV or IM. Nor should the sites of injection be exercised or massaged as suggested for R. Speeding up the action of these other insulins would defeat the purpose of using them. This restriction also applies to mixtures of R with other insulins.

The Cumulative Effect of Injected Insulin

The effect whereby a small portion of injected insulin is temporarily inactivated, only to become available at some unpredictable later time, was mentioned in item 2 on pages 111 and 113. This effect is such a frequent cause of unanticipated hypoglycemia, that it warrants special mention in this chapter.

After a period of experimentation, most patients on our regimen find that their basic daily insulin dosage has stabilized and rarely requires major adjustment. This stabilized dosage, usually requiring 3 or more daily injections, already takes into account the temporary inactivation and later release of some of the injected insulin. One or two additional units of R, on some days, to lower elevated BG, should not cause significant problems.

What if dietary indiscretion, infection, or some other factor causes BG to rise to 400 mg/dl? The typical Type Ia patient may require perhaps 12 units of R over and above the stabilized daily dosage to return BG to normal. If approximately ¼ of these 12 units, or 3 units, are temporarily inactivated and released later, we might observe a delayed BG drop of 3 units $\times$ (30 mg/dl per unit) = 90 mg/dl. If the patient had, using the R, brought his BG down to 100 mg/dl, he might suffer a further drop, many hours later, to $100 - 90$ = 10 mg/dl. The result, of course, is severe hypoglycemia.

The same dire effect can occur if a patient experiences several slight BG elevations during the day and takes several small extra doses of R. The delayed action of the extra doses can be cumulative and possibly cause severe hypoglycemia during the night.

Thus we have yet another reason for careful adherence to diet. Maintenance of normal BG and the use of small total daily insulin doses are essential wherever possible.

Two More Possible Benefits of Physiologic Insulin Dosage

After years of overwhelming evidence, segments of the medical community are finally coming to the conclusion that elevated BG causes the long-term complications of diabetes (see Chapter 2 and Appendix D). Evidence now beginning to accumulate leads us to suspect that the supraphysiologic (unnaturally large) doses of insulin used to treat many diabetics may also be harmful. Aside from the fact that nonphysiologic use of insulin leads to wild fluctuation of BG, we have at least the following two additional situations:

1. Vascular smooth muscle (a tissue in the walls of arteries) is especially susceptible to the anabolic (tissue-building) effects of insulin. High levels of insulin have been found, in tissue culture, to correlate with proliferation of vascular smooth muscle cells. It happens that one of the key stages in the development of atherosclerotic plaques (hardening of arteries) involves proliferation of vascular smooth muscle. Since vascular disease involving such proliferation is commonplace among uncontrolled diabetics, unnecessary use of high insulin doses may accelerate this form of degeneration.

2. Receptor sites for insulin have recently been located in the arcuate nucleus of the hypothalamus, a portion of the brain concerned with feeding behavior (appetite). Since hypoglycemia is known to cause a feeling of starvation that often leads to overeating, it also seems possible that excessive use of insulin will stimulate this appetite center, even when BG is elevated. Perhaps this is part of the reason why so many insulin-dependent diabetics are chronically hungry and overeat even when BG is high.

Trading Units for Minutes

Sooner or later, many patients who monitor BG discover variations on insulin usage that seem to circumvent some of the inconveniences of their usual routines. One of these shortcuts, although it may be of value, also introduces a risk that can be avoided.

Frequently, under social pressure, a diabetic will feel obliged to begin a meal within a few minutes of the pre-prandial dose of Regular insulin, even though the most appropriate "physiologic" behavior might be to delay eating for 30–75 minutes. Ordinarily, the result of such action is an elevated postprandial BG that will continue to increase until treated with additional R. The shortcut is to increase the *preprandial* dose of R by 1 or 2 units in the hope of preventing, or at least minimizing, both the magnitude and the extent in time of the *postprandial* BG increase. However, considerable experimentation is required to determine how much insulin will cover a given change in meal timing. The risk lies in the temptation to take more than is necessary and thereby to precipitate eventual hypoglycemia.

Insulin Usage and the Individual Patient

The many suggestions for insulin regimens that have been set forth in this chapter are *merely guidelines*. Each patient should have a customized regimen that suits individual needs. The insulin regimen should be changed in accord with BG measurements, and not rigidly maintained if inappropriate. When a patient first begins a new regimen, he should be in telephone contact with his physician, at least daily, for the first 1–2 weeks.

The new insulin regimen recommended in this manual, taken alone, will not achieve much for the patient. The entire treatment scheme must be embarked upon simultaneously, if normal BG levels are to be rapidly attained. Therefore, the patient must:

1. Start the new diet (Chapter 13) at the same time as the insulin regimen.

2. Measure BG according to the schedule set forth on page 101.

3. Maintain proper Data Sheets.

4. Treat even slightly elevated BG levels with small doses of R having a known BG-lowering effect.

5. Avoid eating a meal or a snack unless BG is in or below the target range and the meal or snack has been covered by a prior injection of R.

The approximate Ultralente dosage schedules recommended in this chapter are much smaller than current clinical practice dictates. Beware of the temptation to start with high doses of UL, NPH, or other prolonged or intermediate insulins, as the net result is likely to be very disturbing. The traditional approach will not work!

13

THE LOW-CARBOHYDRATE/HIGH-
PROTEIN DIET

SUMMARY

The major sources of dietary energy (calories) and their effects upon blood glucose are as follows:

Fats—not converted to glucose.

Monosaccharides (simple sugars)—rapidly increase BG.

Oligosaccharides (molecular chains of up to ten simple sugars)—raise BG rapidly but more slowly than simple sugars.

Polysaccharides (starches)—increase of BG begins in about 10 minutes but continues for about 1½ hours.

Proteins (from meat, fish, eggs, milk products)—partially converted to BG over a period of about 4 hours.

The diet here recommended seeks to prevent postprandial BG rise entirely, by eliminating the simple sugars and most oligosaccharides, minimizing the use of polysaccharides, and maximizing the slowly utilized proteins. At the same time, we try to minimize saturated and total fats because high fat levels in the blood can predispose to arterial and heart diseases. The diet described in this chapter has succeeded both in normalizing BG and in lowering blood lipid (fat) levels.

Also described is a simplified approach to meal planning which is much more acceptable to patients and eliminates the traditional complex computations involving calories and grams of fat, carbohydrate, and protein.

The topics covered include:

1. Fats.
2. Carbohydrates.
3. Proteins.
4. Alcohol.
5. The timing of dietary effects on BG.
6. The low-carbohydrate/high-protein diet.
7. A simplified approach to meal planning.
8. Possible increases in dietary complex carbohydrate after initial stabilization.
9. Reading labels.
10. Supplementary vitamins and minerals.
11. Artificial sweeteners and diet foods.
12. Dietary fiber.
13. Some considerations regarding dietary fat levels.
14. Comparison of dietary allowances recommended by the American Diabetes Association (ADA) with a typical GLUCOGRAF low-carbohydrate/high-protein diet.
15. Eating away from home.
16. Patient reactions to the new diet.

An essential supplement to this chapter is Appendix A, The GLUCOGRAF List of Food Exchanges for Diabetics. Immediately after reading this chapter, it would be wise to study Appendix A—especially the text that accompanies the various food lists.

Every individual requires outside sources of energy or fuel for survival. These energy sources appear in the diet in the form of carbohydrates, proteins, and fats. A less common source of energy, not in every diet, is alcohol. Most foods contain one or more of these energy sources but every form of food energy affects BG differently. We will now briefly examine each of these basic energy sources.

Fats

Fats are the most concentrated energy sources of all foodstuffs and serve primarily for energy storage. They are found in milk products, cheeses, nuts, oils, and meats. Frequently a food will contain fat in combination with carbohydrate and protein. Every gram of fat contains 9 calories of energy. If the body has no immediate use for this energy, the fat will be stored as body fat until it is needed.

The digestion of fats does not have any direct effect upon BG. From the point of view of BG, diabetics can theoretically eat all the fat they want. In practice, however, large amounts of any food (including fat) will cause the secretion of counter-regulatory enteric hormones into the bloodstream with resultant increase of BG (see Chapter 5). Excessive consumption of fat will, moreover, cause weight gain and can raise the levels of certain fatty substances in the blood. Since these fatty substances might increase the risk of blood vessel disease or coronary heart disease, we usually try to limit dietary fats to less than 40 percent of daily calories.

There is reason to believe that certain types of fats (saturated fats) are more conducive to blood vessel diseases than are other types (polyunsaturated fats). Although the evidence of this is still open to question, the American Heart Association and the American Diabetes Association both urge that polyunsaturated fats be substituted for saturated fats whenever possible. It is believed that the ratio of polyunsaturated fat calories to saturated fat calories (P/S ratio) may be more important than the total amount of fat in the diet. Current practice is to recommend for most adult diabetics a P/S ratio of 1:1 to 1.5:1. This is three to five times greater than the estimated P/S ratio in the average American diet. Nevertheless, some investigators have even recommended dietary P/S ratios greater than 3:1. Familiarity with reference No. 4 in Appendix F, and with the labeling of packaged foods, will enable you to distinguish between saturated fats (usually from animal sources) and polyunsaturated fats (available from certain vegetable sources).

Carbohydrates

Carbohydrates (CHO) are the principal source of energy in most diets throughout the world, simply because carbohydrates are the most readily available and least expensive dietary constituents. Most populations, therefore, consume more carbohydrate than either fat or protein. Carbohydrates are the principal caloric constituents of fruits, many vegetables, confections, soups, bread, most desserts, packaged snacks, crackers, pasta, fruit juices, etc. One gram of carbohydrate contains 4 calories of energy.

A carbohydrate molecule is built up from one or more sugar molecules which are linked together to form the carbohydrate. Carbohydrates are also called saccharides (meaning "sweets"). They may be classified according to the following scheme:

Monosaccharides. Carbohydrates consisting of only one sugar unit. Also called simple sugars.

Oligosaccharides. Carbohydrates consisting of from two to ten sugar units linked together.

Polysaccharides. Carbohydrates consisting of more than ten sugar units linked together. The molecules of some polysaccharides, such as starch, may be made from thousands of sugar units and are therefore very large compared to oligosaccharides. Glycogen is a polysaccharide synthesized in the body for storing small amounts of carbohydrate in liver and muscle. Most carbohydrates found in nature are large polysaccharides. Polysaccharides are also called complex sugars.

Carbohydrates can be formed from many different monosaccharide sugars. For our purposes, two of these sugars are of special interest:

Glucose. Also called D-glucose or dextrose, this monosaccharide is the principal fuel of most organisms and also the building block of the most abundant polysaccharides. In untreated diabetes, the body is unable to properly utilize this basic sugar. In humans, most other sugars or carbohydrates must somehow be converted to glucose by the body, if they are to serve as fuels. Glucose is found in many plants and fruits.

Fructose. Also called "fruit sugar." Found in honey and in most fruits. Like glucose, it is a monosaccharide. Its structure is different from that of glucose, but when blood insulin is absent or at a low level, the body converts fructose to glucose in the liver.

There are three oligosaccharides that are also of special interest:

Sucrose. Consists of one glucose molecule linked to one fructose molecule. It is produced by sugar cane and sugar beets, is abundant in plants and serves as the common sweetener known as table sugar. Sucrose is called a disaccharide because it can be split into two sugar units.

Maltose. Another disaccharide. Consists of two linked glucose molecules. It is formed in the body by the breakdown of starch or other polysaccharides. This breakdown first occurs in the mouth when starchy foods are chewed. The enzyme, amylase, contained in saliva, mixes with the more complex carbohydrates, breaking them down to the two-sugar structure of maltose. When maltose is then swallowed and reaches the small intestine, it is further broken down to glucose by the enzyme maltase.

Lactose. A dissacharide, consisting of a glucose molecule linked to another simple sugar called galactose. Lactose is present in small amounts in milk and is therefore called "milk sugar." Some of the lactose that reaches the intestine is broken down to glucose and galactose by the enzyme lactase.

Most ingested lactose is absorbed directly into the blood-stream and eventually reaches the liver where it is further digested or transformed.

Thus, carbohydrates have different degrees of complexity. Those built from glucose units are converted to glucose somewhere along the digestive process. Glucose is usually absorbed into the bloodstream (as blood sugar) through the walls of the small intestine. The time required for a given carbohydrate to raise BG depends upon how rapidly it is processed to glucose. Most simple sugars raise BG rapidly. More complex sugars and fructose take longer. Some complex carbohydrates are converted to simple sugars merely by cooking. For example, the longer potato (a starchy vegetable) is cooked, the more simple sugars it will contain and the faster, once eaten, it will raise BG.

Fiber is another form of carbohydrate which, if uncooked, has very little effect upon BG. It is actually a group of many different polysaccharides, found in plants, and includes cellulose, hemicellulose, and certain gums. Cellulose, for example, is a polysaccharide found as a component of celery, lettuce, and a number of other vegetables. Cellulose consists of many glucose units, bound together, with linkages that cannot be broken by human digestive enzymes. Thus, cellulose, although a carbohydrate, cannot be digested by humans. (A small fraction of ingested cellulose can be converted to glucose by bacteria in the intestines.) When cellulose molecules leave the human body they are virtually unchanged. Cooking will break many of these linkages and will permit much of the cellulose to be digested. The following vegetables contain much of their carbohydrate as cellulose, and, if uncooked and eaten in reasonable quantities, will have negligible effect upon BG:

Chicory	Lettuce	Watercress
Chinese cabbage	Mushrooms	Others: (See Appendix A, last
Endive	Parsley	two sections of the list of
Escarole	Radish	Vegetable Products)

If the glucose formed by digestion from most carbohydrates is not immediately used for energy, it will be stored by the liver as glycogen, provided that insulin is present. Excess glucose is also converted to precursors of fats called triglycerides. Triglycerides can eventually become incorporated into fatty tissue.

Proteins

Most of the diverse tissues in the bodies of animals, fish, and humans are formed from proteins. Proteins are large molecules, consisting of chains of smaller molecules called amino acids. Muscles, enzymes, certain hormones, and more than 50 percent of the dry mass of the average cell in the body are made of protein. Plants usually contain much smaller proportions of proteins than do animals. Proteins serve principally as structural elements, functional elements, and sources of genetic information, within a living creature. Unlike fats and carbohydrates, proteins are not usually major sources of fuel. In prehistoric times, however, certain carnivorous human or prehuman populations may have consumed protein as the major dietary energy source. One gram of protein contains 4 calories of energy. Our principal dietary sources of protein are meat, fowl, fish, eggs, and cheese.

The amino acids, derived from protein, can be partly converted to glucose by the liver (gluconeogenesis). Individuals with inadequate blood insulin levels may even break down some of their own tissue proteins to amino acids, which are then converted to glucose. This uncontrolled breakdown of protein to glucose is one of the reasons for the great difficulty that poorly controlled juvenile diabetics have in building muscle bulk.

Dietary protein is digested, by intestinal enzymes, to its amino acid building blocks. The amino acids are absorbed into the bloodstream through the intestinal walls. Once in the blood, the amino acids may be used for the construction of new proteins, provided an adequate level of insulin is present. If more protein is digested than is required for new protein construction, the excess is converted to glucose. This new glucose can then be used immediately for energy or can, if adequate insulin is present, be converted to glycogen and stored in the liver and muscles for future energy needs.

The process of digesting protein and then converting the excess amino acids to glucose can require a number of hours for completion. For this reason the direct effect of protein foods on BG, in a properly insulinized individual, is even slower than the effect of complex carbohydrates. There is, however, a secondary effect on BG that can occur quite rapidly during a protein meal, in diabetics who are inadequately supplied with insulin. The absorption of amino acids through the walls of the small intestine can trigger an outpouring into the bloodstream of enteroglucagon, and enteric hormones that stimulate pancreatic A-cells to secrete glucagon (see Chapter 5). The glucagon and enteroglucagon, of course, can cause a rapid increase in BG, which may be unopposed in Type I patients by endogenous insulin. Thus, when a patient has *inadequate blood insulin levels,* there are usually two phases of BG elevation from the eating of proteins:

Phase 1. A rapid BG rise due to glucagon release. Phase I glucagon release can also occur in response to any foods (fats, for example) that cause considerable distention of the small intestine. This usually requires, for example, at least 4 ounces of meat or cheese to become measurable.

Phase 2. A long-term BG rise, over a period of perhaps 2–4 hours, in adults, due to the conversion of amino acids to glucose.

The timing of Phase 2, for many patients, corresponds to the action of small doses of subcutaneously injected Regular insulin. Thus, if a Type I diabetic (with a normal BG) is hungry between meals, he can probably consume a few slices of cheese, then promptly take 1 or 2 units of Regular insulin and experience no change in BG. Similarly, a Type II patient can usually snack without any extra insulin, provided the amount of protein consumed is not excessive. A patient who measures BG can easily determine the amounts of protein, with or without insulin, that he can consume without experiencing any BG rise. Type I patients can similarly determine the requisite insulin dose for a given snack.

Alcohol

Alcohol is a source of energy, in that each gram contains about 7 calories, of which about 5 calories can be utilized by the body. It has no direct effect upon BG but can cause an important secondary effect, which is mentioned below. Many alcoholic beverages, however, do contain substantial amounts of carbohydrate. These additional carbohydrates can significantly raise BG. An 8-ounce glass of beer typically contains 10 grams of carbohydrate or about three-quarters the carbohydrate in a slice of bread.

Alcohol can block gluconeogenesis in the liver. An alcoholic drink near mealtime can prevent the conversion to glucose of all, or part, of amino acids from protein foods. Since our regimen will be using protein as the principal source of dietary glucose, the net result of an alcoholic drink at mealtime can be very dangerous. A portion of the dose of Regular insulin, taken before a meal, is intended to cover the effects of protein on BG. If the protein is not converted to glucose, this insulin can lower BG too far and severe hypoglycemia (insulin reaction) can result. Since the effect of alcohol on the brain can cause a mental confusion similar to that experienced during hypoglycemia, the patient may think that he is only displaying the effects of alcohol when he also is suffering from low BG. Therefore, for patients on our regimen, alcohol can be very dangerous, especially if consumed within three hours of a meal.

The Timing of Dietary Effects on BG

The preceding discussion shows that, for the body to derive glucose from a food, the food must contain either carbohydrate or protein or both. We would anticipate that some
types of foods will be converted to glucose more rapidly than
others. As a result some of these foods will cause a rapid rise
in BG and others will cause a slow rise.

Foods which cause an almost immediate BG increase cannot be adequately covered by Regular insulin, which, when
injected subcutaneously, may exert its maximum effect
within a 3-hour period. The result of consuming such foods is
postprandial BG elevation. If it were not for this effect, Type
I diabetes would be much easier to control and our regimen
would be unnecessary. Not only are these transient high BG
levels likely to increase the long-term likelihood of blood
vessel diseases and other complications, but they are very
difficult to bring down to normal without large doses of insulin. This is because of the resistance to insulin when BG is
elevated. The use of these large, nonphysiologic insulin doses
then leads to hypoglycemia. The resultant hypoglycemia can
occur for a variety of reasons of which two are of special
interest:

1. A large dose of Regular insulin before a meal will produce a very sharp peak of insulin in the blood, which will
usually begin within 45 minutes to 1½ hours. Most patients
will have great difficulty in beginning their meal at *exactly*
the right time to prevent hypoglycemia yet not develop BG
elevation. On the other hand, a small preprandial dose of
Regular insulin produces a broad, shallow blood insulin level
response that can easily be matched to mealtime—even if
eating is unexpectedly delayed for perhaps a half-hour. The
allowable delay for any patient can be determined experimentally with the aid of BG measurement (pages 126–127).

2. We have already indicated (pages 111 and 113) that a

small portion of injected insulin becomes bound to serum or tissue proteins that temporarily inactivate it, but eventually release it with unpredictable timing. Let's follow the hypothetical case of a patient who finds that 1 unit of insulin lowers his BG by 30 mg/dl. Suppose that in this patient one-sixth of all injected Regular insulin is temporarily inactivated. If, before a meal, he administers 6 units of Regular, he can expect that sooner or later 1/6 × 6 units or 1 unit will lower his BG unexpectedly by 30 mg/dl—from perhaps 100 mg/dl to 70 mg/dl. But what happens if he takes 12 units of Regular, to cover a meal that would otherwise rapidly raise BG? The delayed effect will be doubled and at some unexpected time his BG might drop 2 × 30 mg/dl = 60 mg/dl (rapidly or slowly) from 100 mg/dl to 40 mg/dl—a truly hypoglycemic level.

Thus it is essential that, at least for Type I diabetes, glucose loading at meals be avoided. Consideration of the following table should suggest how this can be accomplished.

Food Type and Conversion Process	Approximate Timing for Digestion, Conversion to Glucose, and Appearance as Increased BG	
	BG Rise Begins	Last Trace of Glucose Appears in Blood
Glucose. No digestion required. Moves directly through stomach and intestinal walls into bloodstream.	2 minutes	½ hour
Fructose (fruit sugar). No digestion required. Moves into bloodstream through intestinal walls. Converted by liver to triose-phosphates, which are also intermediate products of glucose metabolism. These will convert to glucose if not covered by additional insulin.	25 minutes	1½ hours

Food Type and Conversion Process	Approximate Timing for Digestion, Conversion to Glucose, and Appearance as Increased BG	
	BG Rise Begins	Last Trace of Glucose Appears in Blood
Sugar alcohols (used as artificial sweeteners, also found in fruits and vegetables). Converted in a manner similar to fructose.	25 minutes	1½ hours
Sucrose (table sugar). Digestion breaks the glucose molecule away from the fructose molecule. The two separate molecules then proceed as above with the original glucose portion appearing as BG first.	5 minutes	1½ hours
Starch and other polysaccharides. Salivary (and pancreatic) amylase breaks down much of it to maltose, which is further degraded to glucose in the small intestine.	10 minutes	1½ hours
Protein. Denatured by acids in stomach, then broken down into amino acids by digestive enzymes in small intestine. Amino acids enter bloodstream and those not used for tissue building are converted to glucose by the liver.	1½ hours (If we ignore the Phase I glucagon effect that can be offset by relatively low blood levels of insulin)	4 hours
Fat. Is not converted to glucose. There does exist a Phase I glucagon effect if consumed in large amounts. This can be offset by relatively low blood levels of insulin.		

From the preceding table we might conclude that the rise in BG after a meal can be slowed considerably by a diet that has the following basic guidelines:

1. No simple sugars or disaccharides such as glucose, fructose, or sucrose. This means no desserts, no fruits, no packaged foods or beverages containing simple sugars.

2. Reduction of polysaccharides (complex carbohydrates), such as starches, to a bare minimum.

3. Replacement of carbohydrate calories by proteins and fats.

These rules, although logical, are a bit too vague and ignore the warnings of the American Heart Association, with respect to fat levels in the diet. Experience with a variety of teenage and adult insulin-dependent patients confirms that the following more precise version of this diet can prevent postprandial glucose elevation, when preceded by *low* doses of Regular insulin. Such a diet can be nutritious, need not be overloaded with fats, and can have a high P/S ratio.

The Low-Carbohydrate/High-Protein Diet

1. No simple sugars or disaccharides such as glucose, fructose, maltose, or sucrose.[1] Therefore no desserts (ice cream, pastries, cookies, etc.), no fruits, no cooked potatoes, and no packaged foods or beverages containing simple sugars or disaccharides. Labels of packaged or canned products may use the legends dextrose, corn syrup solids, etc., to designate certain simple sugars.

Simple sugars may be used for treating insulin reactions, since it is then desirable to raise BG rapidly. Small calibrated amounts of simple sugars or disaccharides (including fruits) may be consumed, while exercising, to prevent hypogly-

---

1. The small amount of lactose found in milk products, although a disaccharide, is converted to glucose at about the same rate as polysaccharides. It is therefore not included in this group of "forbidden" sugars.

11112111

cemia. The procedures for these uses appear in Chapters 14 and 15.

Test strips for urine glucose, such as TES-TAPE (more convenient) (Eli Lilly & Co.) and DIASTIX (more expensive; Ames Co.) are useful for testing soups, sauces, etc. in restaurants. A food product that produces a reaction of no more than 0.5 percent on the test strip probably has a negligibly low level of simple sugars. Most packaged and restaurant soups contain considerable amounts of simple sugars or sucrose. Even soups prepared at home from fresh vegetables may contain high glucose levels if cooked for several hours.

2. Reduce the consumption of polysaccharides to the maximum level that will permit a normal preprandial BG to remain constant after a meal, when the preprandial dose of Regular insulin is about 1/5 of the total daily insulin requirement (Chapter 12). This may involve experimentation over a number of days to determine how much carbohydrate (CHO) can be tolerated in a meal without elevation of BG. Ideally, BG should be the same after ½ hour, 1 hour, 2 hours, 3 hours, and 4 hours, as it was before eating. For Type Ia (no endogenous insulin) adult patients weighing up to 150 pounds, this usually means no more than about 12 grams of CHO per meal. This is the amount of CHO in one bread exchange [2] or in one glass of milk. Type Ib and Type II patients may be able to tolerate more CHO, but the amount must be determined by experiment.

3. It is probably wise to minimize the consumption of fats, especially the saturated fats. This is a general recommenda-

---

2. The "bread exchange" is the basic unit of measure that we use for complex carbohydrate in our diet. It is based on the common 23-gram slice and *contains 12 grams of CHO*. This manual does not use the American Diabetes Association bread exchange, which is based upon a 27-gram slice and contains 15 grams of CHO. All carbohydrate-containing foods listed in Appendix A are shown with their CHO content in grams and the equivalent bread exchange value.

tion that applies even to nondiabetics and does not relate to the control of BG. As it turns out, a fair amount of fat will come into the diet in the protein portions, since all meats, fishes, whole milk, and cheeses contain some fat. (The list of protein food products in Appendix A is broken down into three groups based on low, intermediate, and high fat content.) One should therefore try to avoid such foods as butter, saturated cooking oils, fried foods, ice cream, egg yolk, whole milk, whole-milk cheeses, etc. Egg white, skim milk, skim-milk cheese products, and safflower cooking oil are good substitutes. Dietary salad dressings that are low in saturated fat and have no more than 2 grams of carbohydrate per serving are readily available in food markets. Remember, however, that for Type I diabetics, loading with carbohydrate will probably be more harmful in the long run than loading with fats. The consequences of poor BG control occur much more rapidly than do the consequences of excessive consumption of saturated fats.

4. The additional calories necessary to maintain ideal body weight, above and beyond the CHO exchanges, should be provided by protein. In all likelihood, the protein calories will exceed both the CHO and fat calories in any given day. Consider the following example:

A patient is eating a 1,500-calorie-per-day diet. The calories are to be distributed equally between three meals. An evening meal might have the following breakdown:

A. A salad containing lettuce, radishes, Chinese cabbage, and similar low-carbohydrate vegetables from sections 5 and 6 of the Vegetable Products list in Appendix A. These vegetables provide vitamins and minerals but, if uncooked, virtually no carbohydrate and no calories.

carbohydrate	1 gram
fat	0 grams
protein	0 grams

B. Two servings (6 teaspoons) of "low-calorie" bleu cheese salad dressing.

carbohydrate	2 grams
fat	2 grams
protein	1 gram

C. One vegetable from the ⅓ bread exchange section of the Vegetable Products list in Appendix A.

carbohydrate	5 grams
fat	0 grams
protein	2 grams

D. 7 ounces of lean meat.

carbohydrate	0 grams
fat	21 grams
protein	49 grams

E. ⅔ glass of skim milk.

carbohydrate	8 grams
fat	0 grams
protein	5 grams

The preceding meal contains a total of:

16 grams carbohydrate	@ 4 calories each =	64
23 grams fat	@ 9 calories each =	207
57 grams protein	@ 4 calories each =	<u>228</u>
Total calories		499

The total of 499 calories is about one-third of the daily diet of 1,500 calories. It contains 13 percent CHO (64 cal. ÷ 499 cal.), 41 percent fat (207 cal. ÷ 499 cal.), and 46 percent protein (228 cal. ÷ 499 cal.).

There could be many variations on this meal. For example, the P/S ratio could have been improved by substituting safflower oil, vinegar, and spices for the low-calorie bleu cheese salad dressing.

An ideal low-carbohydrate/high-protein diet might contain, in the average meal: 15 percent carbohydrate calories, at least 45 percent protein calories, and no more than 40 percent fat calories. This would be for a Type Ia patient. Patients with significant C-peptide levels may tolerate more CHO.

There are available in the U.S.A. several foods high in protein and low in carbohydrate and saturated fats, which the author has found of considerable value in his personal diet. These include:

1. Broiled swordfish (low fat).

2. White meat turkey without skin (low fat, mostly poly-unsaturated).

3. EGGBEATERS ® (Standard Brands, Inc., 625 Madison Avenue, New York, N.Y. 10022). Each 8-ounce package contains 28 grams protein, 12 grams CHO, and no fat. Made from egg whites (egg yolks have high cholesterol content).

4. Tunafish, canned, water-packed (only a trace of fat).

5. Sturgeon, smoked (very little fat, but expensive).

6. CHEEZOLA ® (Fisher Cheese Co., Wapakoneta, Ohio 45895). 50 percent protein, 50 percent fat with a P/S ratio of 4:1. Resembles ordinary process cheese but is made from skim milk and corn oil. Inexpensive, tasty, and sold by mail order.

7. The following low-fat cheeses contain less than 3 grams of fat per ounce and virtually no CHO:
LITE LINE pasteurized process cheese (Borden)
SLIM LINE pasteurized process cheese (Swift)
Skim American (Borden)
Tilset-Slim (imported)
Weight Watchers low-fat cheese slices
CALORIE WISE cheese spread (Kraft)
TASTY LOAF cheese spread (Kraft)

Additional protein products with low fat content are listed in Appendix A.

A Simplified Approach to Meal Planning

The conventional approach to custom-tailoring meal plans for individual diabetics has been complex and possibly more difficult for patients to comprehend and remember than our insulin, diet, and blood glucose regimens combined. It involves computation of a patient's ideal body weight (IBW); computation of the calories required to maintain IBW; computation of calorie addition or subtraction so that IBW can be reached; conversion of daily calories to grams of fat, protein, and carbohydrate; conversion of grams to fat exchanges, meat exchanges, milk exchanges, vegetable exchanges, and so on. Most of the computations, some of which resemble those on pages 157–158, are performed by dietitians, and all of the memorization must be done by the patient or the patient's family.

With our simplified approach, the patient can work out his/her own meal plan and must remember only a few simple rules. The key to our simplified approach will be a scale. We ask that every patient own a scale—not the kind for weighing food (although that is also worth having), but the kind that weighs people. We then proceed as follows:

1. The patient is advised of the total number of bread exchanges of complex CHO prescribed for a meal—usually one bread exchange per meal for nonpregnant, adult, or teenage Type Ia patients. Somewhat more CHO is feasible for Type Ib, Type II or some pregnant patients.

2. The patient is instructed to take approximately the same dose of Regular insulin prior to each of 3 meals, so that the amount of CHO and protein can be kept essentially the same for each meal. Fats can vary from meal to meal because they are not converted to glucose. We therefore do not oblige the patient to eat a predetermined amount of fat.

3. In addition to the complex CHO, the patient should consume enough protein to satisfy hunger, but not enough to cause BG elevation at any time within 4 hours of the meal.

Extra-saturated fats (for example, butter, cream, egg yolks, etc.) should be avoided, since most low-fat protein products (see Appendix A, pages 228 and 229) will also bring some saturated fats to the diet.

4. The physician should advise the patient of a plan for weight loss, weight gain, or weight maintenance. By "plan" we mean pounds per week to be gained/lost, or alternately no weight change.

5. The patient should weigh himself/herself every 2 or 3 days at the same hour.

   a. If weight is according to plan, then the diet needn't be changed.

   b. If weight is too high, then protein and any accompanying fats (as in meat and cheese) should be reduced slightly in future meals. It may also be necessary to reduce the doses of Regular insulin by very small amounts—perhaps by ½ unit at a time. Alternately, a patient may wish to eliminate one or more meals per week and also eliminate the dose of Regular insulin that would have preceded those meals.

   c. If weight is too low, then protein, and any accompanying fat, should be increased. This may require slight increases in preprandial doses of Regular insulin. Such increases should initially be small—perhaps only ½ unit at a time. Polyunsaturated fats may also be added to meals.

6. If weight is appropriate, BG remains normal, and patient is still hungry at the end of a meal, he should try increasing his intake of salads [3] prepared from any of the following

---

3. The value of salad as a nutritious, hunger-satisfying adjunct to our low-CHO diet cannot be overemphasized. Many diabetics who rarely ate salads became addicted to them after starting our regimen. The key lay frequently in the selection of salad dressings. Some people rapidly settle on one type of dressing, while others sample every new dressing that they see in the supermarket, and keep collections of different dressings in their kitchens. One large salad, complete with several tablespoons of dressing, frequently contains less CHO than the one bread exchange allocated to most meals. Furthermore, the high fiber content of many uncooked vegetables may slow the absorption of the CHO that they contain (see pages 167–171).

raw vegetables, which contain very little available carbohydrate, protein, or fat:

Chicory	Lettuce	Watercress
Chinese cabbage	Mushrooms	Others—(see Appendix A,
Endive	Parsley	sections 5 and 6 of the list
Escarole	Radishes	of Vegetable Products)

Care should be taken not to overeat. Excessive distention of the small intestine can cause an outpouring of glucagon that will raise BG.

By maintaining body weight at the prescribed level, the patient is automatically consuming the proper number of daily calories. He will be less likely to experience hunger between meals because his high-protein diet is digested very slowly. He is freer to experiment and is less dependent upon professionals for instruction on dietary modifications. He is also more likely to learn about new sources of protein, polyunsaturated fats, etc., especially if he consults his handbooks (this manual, Appendix A, and Reference 4, Appendix E) and reads labels on packaged foods.

Possible Increases in Dietary Complex Carbohydrate After Initial BG Stabilization

The dietary guidelines of the preceding section probably encompass the maximum amount of CHO that fully insulin-dependent (Type Ia) patients can tolerate without eliciting substantial BG disturbances. Diabetics who are producing significant amounts of endogenous insulin (Type Ib and Type II) can probably tolerate diets with more calories coming from complex CHO. Such diets can offer at least three advantages to the patient:

1. CHO is less expensive than protein, calorie for calorie.

2. CHO calories are readily available without the presence of fat.

3. Additional CHO can add more variety to any diet.

4. Additional CHO offers the opportunity to add grains (important sources of B-complex vitamins) to the diet without the need for vitamin supplements or lots of green vegetables.

It is therefore suggested that once a Type Ib or Type II diabetic has attained normal BG at least 90 percent of the time and has fully normalized HbA_{1c}, he/she might experiment with gradually increasing the CHO content of a meal while reducing the protein content. This should be done one meal at a time and should involve small increments in complex CHO, no greater than ½ bread exchange (6 grams CHO) at a time. It is a good opportunity to introduce grains (bread, cereals, rice) into the diet. Postprandial BG should be monitored carefully. It is possible that Type Ib patients may have to increase their preprandial doses of Regular insulin. In most cases such increases will be *less than* one unit R for every additional ½ bread exchange. Protein intake should be reduced by 2 grams for every added gram of CHO—otherwise the added calories will cause weight gain.

Remember that the main reason for keeping dietary CHO low was to minimize the dosage of R. Low doses, up to perhaps 4 units per meal for Type Ib patients, permit some flexibility in the amount of time between injecting insulin and starting the meal. Higher doses can make timing so critical that the inconvenience and hazard of hypoglycemia may not justify the added CHO.

Reading Labels

It is important that patients and their families develop the habit of reading the nutrition information on the labels of prepared foods, with a special eye to carbohydrate content. The following hints may be of value to the novice:

1. Products that list the number of grams of carbohydrate, protein, and fat per serving are safer than those which list

ingredients but do not have a quantitative breakdown.

2. Note the stated size of one serving. This is frequently different from what the consumer may consider a satisfactory serving.

3. Ingredient names ending in "ose," such as xylose, mannose, dextrose, glucose, sucrose, fructose, etc., are usually sugars.

4. Ingredient names ending in "ol," such as sorbitol, mannitol, xylitol, etc., are usually sugar alcohols and affect BG about as rapidly as polysaccharides (complex sugars).

5. "Corn syrup" or "corn syrup solids" are composed principally of fructose or fructose and glucose.

6. In the U.S. ingredients are listed in order of their percentage in the product, if actual percentages are not shown. Thus, if a label shows dextrose as the third of ten ingredients, the product is probably loaded with sugar, while a label with dextrose as the tenth ingredient probably indicates a negligible amount of sugar.

7. Most packaged soups and sauces contain large amounts of sugar.

Supplementary Vitamins and Minerals

Supplementary vitamins and minerals should be used with caution as excessive quantities can inhibit the body's own synthesis of certain vitamins and intestinal absorption of certain minerals. Poorly controlled diabetics usually put out a large daily volume of urine and thus spill much of their water-soluble vitamins and minerals. It is, therefore, common practice to prescribe therapeutic doses of vitamin and mineral supplements for such patients. Patients on our regimen, once properly regulated, should rarely show urine glucose and therefore will not be urinating excessively. Such patients do not, usually, need vitamin and mineral supplements, if they eat a variety of vegetables. One possible exception results from our virtual elimination of breads and grains. Since these products are major sources of B-complex vitamins, it may be wise to add a daily B-complex capsule, or to eat some bean sprouts, spinach, broccoli, brussels sprouts, or cauliflower each day. This subject is discussed further in Appendix A.

Artificial Sweeteners and Diet Foods

At the time of printing this manual, there is only one artificial sweetener on the market in the U.S. that contains no carbohydrates; it is called saccharin.[3] Researchers, administering very large daily doses of saccharin to laboratory rats, were recently successful in increasing the incidence of bladder cancer in these animals. The doses of saccharin used would be equivalent to feeding humans each day the amount of saccharin in 800 bottles of diet soft drinks. Diabetics have been consuming relatively large amounts of saccharin for many years, yet the incidences of various forms of cancer are not different among diabetics from those among nondiabetics. Both the American Diabetes Association (ADA) and the Juvenile Diabetes Foundation consider saccharin to be safe for consumption by diabetics in the light of present evidence. A more pleasant-tasting sweetener, calcium cyclamate, is still available in some countries.

Many other sweeteners are being marketed as dietary or low-calorie products. At present, at least in the U.S., all such products contain carbohydrate—in the forms of either simple or complex sugars or sugar alcohols. Federal law, in the U.S., requires that these sugars be named on product labels, but often the print size is so small as to be barely legible. One very popular product, called SWEET 'N LOW ®, is designated by the manufacturer as a "sugar substitute." The con-

---

3. It is conceivable that other noncaloric sweeteners, such as ASPARTAME ™ (G.D. Searle), might be approved by the Food and Drug Administration for sale in the U.S.A. at some time in the future.

tents are printed in pale red ink, 50 characters to the inch, on pink paper. With the aid of a magnifying glass, one can discern that the product is 94 percent dextrose (glucose). This product and others can be designated as "sugar free" or "sugar substitute" because, in the U.S., the food-labeling laws identify "sugar" as sucrose. Glucose, fructose, maltose, ribose, mannose, etc., are not legally "sugar."

It is, therefore, especially important to read carefully the labels of any products intended for dietary use. With the exception of some saccharin-sweetened soft drinks, gelatins, and syrups, virtually all such products contain high levels of carbohydrate.

Dietetic pastries, fruit preserves, ice creams, and the like should be avoided—even if sweetened with saccharin. The flour used in pastry and the fruits used in preserves are carbohydrate products. The addition of saccharin does not remove starches or fructose. Furthermore, many "dietetic" foods contain enough simple sugars to raise BG faster than it can be covered by additional R.

Recently, fructose has been promoted as an ideal sweetener for diabetics because it is "metabolized more slowly than sugar." Nevertheless, fructose is still a carbohydrate and must be covered by insulin like any other carbohydrate.

Dietary products advertised in publications of the American Diabetes Association are not necessarily recommended by that organization; nor are such products tested for carbohydrate content. For example, a recent issue of their popular journal, *Diabetes Forecast*, advertises "sugar-free" gum drops, frozen blueberries with "no sugar added," and "the ultimate in confections [candies] for the Diabetic," containing "no salt" and "no saccharin." Although all of these advertisements may comply with U.S. laws, the products are principally carbohydrate (usually fructose or sorbitol) and are best avoided by insulin-dependent patients. Furthermore, the sugar alcohols, sorbitol, mannitol, and xylitol, used to sweeten the candy products, draw water into the bowel and can cause diarrhea when eaten in moderate to large amounts.

Nevertheless, sorbitol, mannitol, xylitol, and fructose affect BG slowly and can be substituted for all or part of the complex carbohydrate at a meal. This may mean trading three vegetable portions for five sorbitol-sweetened gumdrops. Is such a trade worthwhile?

Dietary Fiber

Several years ago, it was noticed that the citizens of modern Western nations suffered from a much higher incidence of cancer of the colon than do primitive tribespeople. It was suggested that the high levels of nonnutritive plant fiber present in primitive diets diluted toxic substances or irritants that might be either present in trace amounts in certain foods or produced during the digestion of nutritive foods.

It was also discovered that some rural populations which consumed diets high in fiber displayed low incidence of diabetes mellitus. This led to research into the possible use of dietary fiber to slow absorption of glucose from carbohydrate foods.

When speculation about the possible advantages of high fiber diets appeared in the popular press, the stimulus for a new type of "fad" diet was generated. One result has been extravagant claims to the effect that the consumption of food containing fiber is inevitably of special benefit to diabetics. There is some evidence that, indeed, a very few special foodstuffs may be of some value. Nevertheless, the *haphazard* consumption of fiber-containing foods can be deleterious to BG control in Type Ia patients.

As mentioned earlier in this section, certain structural polysaccharides, found in plants such as cellulose and gums, if uncooked, cannot be digested to glucose by humans. After

consumption, some fibrous polysaccharides absorb considerable amounts of water, become bulky, and pass through the
intestines too rapidly for complete digestion to occur. Other
types of fiber slow the intestinal transit time, thereby slowing
digestion of all foods, including carbohydrates. The net result
may be a reduction in postprandial BG elevation, especially
in non-insulin-dependent patients.

A practical problem is that the most effective of these
substances, guar gum and pectin, are not readily available in
concentrated palatable form. Actually these two substances
are not fibrous and are more properly classified as unabsorbable carbohydrates. Guar and pectin form gels in the presence
of water, the guar gel being especially sticky and difficult to
swallow. Guar powder, which is particularly effective, must
be baked into bread or somehow added to other foods. Both
substances appear to be effective only when mixed with the
CHO that is to be "slowed." This severely limits their practical application. Typical successful doses of guar powder are
in the range of 5–8 grams per meal.

There is also evidence that guar, pectin, and some other
high-fiber products may bring about reduction in serum cholesterol levels. The fiber does this by binding bile acids
which, in turn are bound to cholesterol. The bile-acid–gum
combination is eliminated from the intestines, thereby lowering total body cholesterol but also depleting the recirculat-
ing bile acid pool. Bile acids are necessary for emulsification
of dietary fats. This depletion leads to inadequate fat digestion, flatulence (expulsion of intestinal gases) and bulky stool.
The high concentration of bile salts in the colon together
with the gum or fiber leads to absorption of water by the
feces, which in turn causes diarrhea. In theory, at least, the
continuous depletion of bile acids can also lead to the formation of cholesterol gallstones.

There are several sources of plant fiber which appear to
bring about some reduction in postprandial BG elevation in

some Type Ib and Type II patients, but do not seem to do so in Type Ia patients. These include:

Soy hulls	Summer squash
Corn bran (not wheat bran)	Zucchini
Celery	

Most high-fiber foods other than seed and bean hulls contain high amounts of absorbable carbohydrate, in addition to the fiber. It is very possible that by *substituting* these high-fiber vegetable products for other vegetables with similar or slightly higher CHO levels, the higher carbohydrate levels can be tolerated. Restricting vegetables to only those on the preceding brief list can interfere with adequate vitamin and mineral nutrition by limiting the variety of vegetables that one might consume over a period of time. A patient monitoring his own BG can experiment with the effects of high fiber foods and unabsorbable carbohydrates. It is unlikely that dramatic results will be secured, except, perhaps, by mixing CHO foods with guar gum, which is not available at retail stores.

It is possible that, at some time in the future, food products may be developed which will, conveniently, improve oral glucose tolerance for Type Ia diabetics. In the meanwhile, a drug developed at Bayer AG in West Germany appears to achieve a similar result by interfering with the enzymatic breakdown of polysaccharides in the gut. This drug, designated BAYg 5421, is being tested on animals in the U.S.A. and on humans abroad. If it has no adverse side effects, it may become available commercially. Its effectiveness, for Type Ia patients, is currently controversial and it may cause unpleasant intestinal disturbances in all "Types" of patients.

Some Considerations Regarding Dietary Fat Levels

One objection, that has been frequently raised, to our low-carbohydrate/high-protein diet, is that any diet high in protein is likely to be high in saturated fats. This is because major sources of proteins are meat and milk products, and animal proteins are usually accompanied by significant quantities of saturated fats. The fat contents of typical diets conforming to our regimen range from 30 to 42 percent of total calories. The current average fat intake of U.S. citizens is now 42 percent of calories, but the U.S. Senate Select Committee on Nutrition and Human Needs now advocates that citizens attempt to reduce this to about 30 percent.

We feel that when it comes to the treatment of insulin-dependent diabetes, our first concern should be prevention of wild BG swings, which can cause immediate danger (hypoglycemia) and many long-term complications. These complications are short term (typically 15–20 years), in comparison to the blood vessel diseases that appear in nondiabetics with sedentary habits and high saturated-fat diets (typically 40–60 years).

Nevertheless, we would like to see diabetics at less cardiovascular risk than the average U.S. citizen. This goal can be pursued with the help of the special protein sources, listed in this chapter, page 159, and in Appendix A (pages 228–231), that contain virtually no saturated fats, supplemented by certain food products that are very high in polyunsaturated fats, such as safflower oil for salad dressings and cooking. Furthermore, we have not yet mentioned strenuous exercise as a factor in protection against cardiovascular diseases. That is covered in Chapter 15. We should point out, however, that exercise reduces blood and tissue levels of certain fats and improves HDL cholesterol levels (pages 64–65). The exercising insulin-dependent diabetic will require frequent ingestion of simple sugars while exercising. This will increase the amount of carbohydrate in the actual diet and thus reduces the real percentage of dietary fat. The fat reduction will usually be fairly small (perhaps 5 percent of total fats).

Comparison of Dietary Breakdown Recommended by the American Diabetes Association with a Typical GLUCOGRAF Low-Carbohydrate/High-Protein Diet

The advocacy of lower carbohydrate intake outlined in this manual deviates from the 1979 recommendations of the American Diabetes Association [4] for a higher CHO intake. Although not specifically stated, this ADA recommendation was probably intended for the majority of diabetics (Type II) who have the ability to produce substantial amounts of insulin. Some patients and health care professionals have been confused by the apparent conflict of goals which may be created for Type I and possibly some Type II patients by the 1979 statement which reiterates a 1976 ADA statement (see Appendix D) stressing the need for normalization of BG to prevent or reduce long-term complications.

	ADA Recommended Dietary Ranges (percent)	Typical GLUCOGRAF Diet, with Extra CHO When Exercising (for Type Ia diabetics) (percent)
Protein	12–20	45
Carbohydrate	50–60	17–25[5]
Fat	30–38	30–38

Why are there such striking differences between the carbohydrate and protein sections of the two approaches to dia-

---

4. American Diabetes Association. Special Report: Principles of Nutrition and Dietary Recommendations for People with Diabetes Mellitus, *Diabetes* 28:1027–1030 (1979).

5. As already indicated on pages 162–163, some Type Ib and Type II patients may be able to maintain normal BG levels with more than 25 percent dietary CHO.

betic diets shown above? Or, more curiously, why does the
ADA recommend high levels of dietary carbohydrate? A
small part of the answer lies in the discovery that some non-
insulin-dependent (Type II) diabetics and nondiabetics produced less insulin in response to a glucose "challenge" when
their dietary carbohydrate was reduced.[6] Subsequent attempts to duplicate this research have both supported and
contradicted the conclusions. Since only about 20 percent of
diabetics are insulin-dependent, little thought was given to
the special needs of the insulin-dependent minority. Furthermore, since the nondiabetic population was already consuming about 45–50 percent carbohydrates, relatively little
dietary modification would be necessary for new diabetics,
and a high level of patient compliance could be anticipated.
The myth that the high doses of insulin used to cover high-
CHO diets are without repercussions probably also played a
role in the decision.

Another important factor was the common belief that the
historic complications found in long-term diabetics were not
due to poor control of BG, but might be in part due to the
high intake of fats, common in the earlier low-carbohydrate
diets.

While this logic may possibly apply to some or even most
Type II diabetics, it certainly conflicts with the physiologic
needs of most insulin-dependent patients. Such patients
should not consume more CHO than is compatible with stabilization of BG at normal levels.

Eating Away from Home

Strangely enough, the temptation of fancy desserts and
starchy foods is not the principal problem encountered by
people on our regimen, when eating at restaurants or at

---

6. Reduced insulin binding over short but not extended time periods has also
been reported.

homes of friends. The more common problems, in sequence of relative importance, appear to be:

1. *Hypoglycemia, due to serving delays and overestimation of Regular insulin needs.* Protein portions at restaurants are frequently even larger than those called for by our high-protein diet. In anticipation of this likelihood, patients would increase their preprandial dose of Regular insulin by 1 or 2 units. They compounded the problem by injecting at home and then traveling to the restaurant or host's home. All too frequently, waiting time at the restaurant was longer than anticipated. Hypoglycemia was the inevitable result. Frequently this problem can be circumvented in the following way: The patient waits until arriving at the restaurant and placing the order before injecting Regular insulin. He injects his usual dose, without any extra. He then waits until the main course is served, estimates the size of the protein portion and, if necessary, administers another 1 or 2 units of insulin. Remember that it takes as long for the protein to be digested as for the Regular insulin to become fully utilized. Efforts at persuading people merely to leave the excess protein on the plate are usually fruitless. It seems that no one wants to waste meat.

2. *High postprandial BG due to large meat portions.* Patients have on occasion not bothered to take the second injection of Regular insulin, just mentioned. Sometimes the logic goes—"Why guess at a dose when I can measure my BG at home, three hours after eating, and perhaps find that I didn't require any extra insulin?" Quite frequently, the resulting BG is very high—perhaps 300–400 mg/dl for Group Ia patients.

3. *Undetected hypoglycemia, after an alcoholic drink.* We have already mentioned in this chapter alcohol's inhibition of gluconeogenesis, and the cerebral effect that can mask hypoglycemia. The only further admonition we can give is, if a patient must drink, he must also be equipped to measure

BG on the spot, even if using the visual/reagent strip method (pages 71; 87–88).

4. *Unsuspected sugar in sauces, salad dressings, soups, and the like.* Discreet use of a small piece of TES-TAPE ® (Lily) will usually detect added sugar. A light green color is usually acceptable; a dark green usually indicates significant amounts of added sugar.

Patient Reactions to the New Diet

Most patients adapt readily to the BG measurements and multiple insulin injections. They inevitably have initial difficulty coping with a diet that forces them to give up desserts, potatoes, pasta, fruit, ice cream, yogurt, peanut butter, and the other high-CHO foods that they have been in the habit of eating. As their BG's approach normal for longer and longer periods, they lose the chronic hunger that plagues most diabetics. Eventually most find that it is more comfortable to eat fewer goodies yet not be hungry than to live to eat but be continually famished.

Many also experience a change in tastes. As they lose their exposure to sweets and junk foods they begin to appreciate salads and low-fat protein products. This transformation of taste takes many months but appears to be fairly common.

Early in the regimen, perplexing BG values are frequently reported. The great bulk of these relate to inappropriate dietary habits such as:

1. Extra protein at dinner, not covered by extra R.
2. Improper timing of a meal relative to the preprandial dose of R.
3. Eating a meal or snack when BG is elevated. This is probably the most common problem. People sometimes think that because they took enough additional preprandial R to lower an elevated BG eventually, they can begin to eat

while BG is still elevated. The nonlinear response of BG to insulin will usually cause a postprandial BG rise that can only be brought down by even more R. Of course, this is a situation that we try to avoid. This rule has an important exception as shown by the following example: Before lunch you had a BG of 225. You therefore injected your usual preprandial dose of 5R plus an extra 4R to bring BG back to normal. After 2¼ hours BG has dropped to 100 mg/dl, so you eat lunch. Before you finish lunch, you have a severe insulin reaction (BG less than 50 mg/dl). Why? Because by the time BG dropped to 100 mg/dl, both doses of insulin (5R and 4R) were entering the blood at a very rapid rate, much faster than digestion could convert the lunch to glucose. In this situation where nearly double the usual preprandial R was administered, you should have eaten when BG was still slightly elevated—perhaps at 130 mg/dl.

At this point it may be helpful to consider Appendix A— The GLUCOGRAF List of Food Exchanges for Diabetics. Carefully read the introduction to each section of the list and become familiar with the list itself.

14

TREATMENT OF HYPOGLYCEMIA
WITHOUT BLOOD GLUCOSE REBOUND

SUMMARY

This chapter lists some of the causes of hypoglycemia and describes a method for correcting low BG without causing BG to rebound to high levels. The reader is taught how to calibrate the effect on BG of a candy, sugar cube, and the like. When hypoglycemia is suspected, the patient measures BG and, if low, takes exactly the number of calibrated sweets required to bring BG back to the target value. Very frequently hypoglycemic symptoms occur and BG is nevertheless found to be normal (explained in the text). Topics covered include:

1. Some causes of unanticipated hypoglycemia.
2. How low must BG be to warrant treatment?
3. The importance of first measuring BG.
4. Using pulse rate as a crude indicator of hypoglycemia.
5. The use of calibrated sweets.
6. Calibration of sweets in BG units.
7. Avoiding BG "overshoot" or rebound when treating hypoglycemia.
8. Treatment when hypoglycemia results in the patient becoming confused or semiconscious.

9. Treating hypoglycemia in the unconscious patient.
10. Treating hypoglycemia after a meal.
11. Impaired sexual functioning when BG is low.

Some Causes of Unanticipated Hypoglycemia

Although one may carefully follow all the dietary, insulin dosage, and BG monitoring techniques presented thus far, it is inevitable that sooner or later BG will fall below the target range and hypoglycemia (inadequate BG, also called insulin reaction) will occur.

The patient should now be in control of the major factors affecting BG, but so many minor factors are encountered every day that many of them will be beyond his/her ability to compensate promptly. Some of these factors are even beyond the ability to predict. Here are a few situations that may bring about unanticipated hypoglycemia:

Unexpected delay of a meal.

Release of that portion of extra insulin doses that has been temporarily bound to antibodies or to inactive sites within body tissues (pages 111 and 113).

Reduced activity of counter-regulatory hormones during certain phases of the menstrual cycle.

Sudden termination of insulin resistance caused by prior illness or stress.

Injecting from a fresh vial of insulin after having used insulin that slowly lost its level of activity over a period of weeks or months.

Underestimation of food portions.

Injection of wrong insulin dose.

Underestimation of physical activity.

Consumption of alcohol prior to a meal.

Failure to vigorously shake vials of modified (cloudy) insulins before use.

Accidental injection of insulin into a muscle or blood vessel.

Injection near a muscle that will be strenuously exercised.

Use of aspirin in large doses, anticoagulants, sulfonamides, barbiturates, antihistamines, or certain other pharmaceuticals that may lower BG. Reference 1 in Appendix E contains a more complete list of drugs that can affect BG.

Most insulin-dependent diabetics and most health care professionals are familiar with the many possible subjective and observable symptoms of hypoglycemia, so these will not be described here. As any patient who monitors BG can attest, hypoglycemia can occur without any discernible sign or symptom (except, perhaps, increased pulse rate). It is therefore not uncommon for a patient to have a BG of 30 mg/dl and not realize that he is hypoglycemic. This problem is compounded by the fact that a slow drop in BG can eventually lower glucose level in the brain to a point where the patient is unable to perceive subtle signs of hypoglycemia.

Patients who follow our regimen, fortunately, will usually experience less frequent and less severe hypoglycemia than patients on more conventional regimens. Furthermore, they are able, upon routine testing, to discover a slightly low BG before glucose level has dropped low enough to produce symptoms.

How Low Must BG Be to Warrant Treatment?

Before we discuss the proper treatment of low BG, we must decide how low it should be permitted to drop before treatment is necessary. In Chapter 12, we arbitrarily estab-

4.4 - 6.8

5, 6

lished a target BG range of 80–120 mg/dl and a target value of 100 mg/dl. Therefore, most patients should raise BG when it drops to about 80–85 mg/dl. This value may be too high during pregnancy, when nondiabetics routinely experience BG levels lower than the usual normal values. The physician may, therefore, wish to permit BG to drop to a low of 65–70 mg/dl before a pregnant patient takes corrective measures. On the other hand, nonpregnant patients, new to this regimen, who have adapted to high BG levels may be very uncomfortable at normal BG values. These patients may have been given an initial target range higher than 80–120 mg/dl, and should raise BG when it reaches the low end of that range. Whatever the assigned range may be, low BG should be raised to the midpoint of that range and no higher. Thus if the range is 80–120 mg/dl, a BG below 80–85 mg/dl should be brought up to 100 mg/dl and no higher.

The Importance of First Measuring BG

At the very first suggestion of hypoglycemic symptoms it is mandatory that the patient measure BG. Without an objective measurement, there is no way of confirming that BG is really low, nor would it be possible to know exactly how much the BG must be raised.

False symptoms of hypoglycemia are not uncommon. After extended periods of chronically elevated BG, the counter-regulatory mechanisms of many diabetics have come to recognize certain elevated BG levels as "normal." Therefore lower, but still elevated BG's cause an outpouring of catecholamines into the blood. These hormones then can cause increased heart rate and other symptoms that mimic hypoglycemia. A patient whose BG chronically exceeds 200 mg/dl may feel hypoglycemic whenever it drops below 150 mg/dl. This can be corrected by slowly lowering his target

BG from perhaps 170 mg/dl to 100 mg/dl over a period of weeks or months.

Ordinary hunger mimics the hunger of hypoglycemia and can trigger other false symptoms of hypoglycemia, by a mechanism that psychologists call a "conditional response." Similarly, anxiety can bring about increased blood levels of catecholamines. The anxiety over such symptoms causes further release of catecholamines and exacerbates the symptoms. Without BG measurement it's a losing battle.

It is therefore very desirable for patients to have their meters with them at all times. Battery-operated meters are particularly valuable because of their portability. At the very least, patients should carry CHEMSTRIP bG strips which can be read by eye as described in Chapters 8 and 9. But remember, hypoglycemic individuals can grossly misread the CHEMSTRIP bG. They are less likely to misuse a reflectance colorimeter.

Using Pulse Rate as a Crude Indicator of Hypoglycemia

If a patient suspects hypoglycemia and has no reagent strips with him, there is a last resort that may be of value. In virtually all patients, resting heart rate (pulse) will increase during hypoglycemia. Usually, the hypoglycemic resting pulse will beat faster than at other times, and (if the patient is conscious) the more severe the hypoglycemia, the faster the pulse. This information can be put to use in the following manner:

1. Every insulin-dependent diabetic should wear a watch with a sweep second hand, at all times. This watch may also be of use for timing BG tests when reagent strips are available.

2. The patient should know his resting pulse rate.

3. The patient must be taught to measure his own pulse rate. The pulse can most easily be found by *very light* finger-

tip pressure at the carotid artery (in groove at sides of throat, just under the "hinge"—joint—of the jawbone) or at the temporal artery (at sides of head above ends of eyebrows). The number of beats is counted for exactly 15 seconds and the result multiplied by 4 to get beats per minute (pulse rate).

4. If the patient suspects hypoglycemia and has no reagent strips with him, he should measure his resting pulse. If it is more than one-third faster than his usual resting pulse, there is a good possibility of hypoglycemia. In a fully conscious patient, a crude rule of thumb would be: the faster the pulse, the lower the BG. Physical activity within 10 minutes prior to measurement can invalidate the result.

The Use of Calibrated Sweets

Low BG, whether with or without symptoms, should be treated immediately, with a calibrated amount of simple sugar, preferably glucose (dextrose) or sucrose (table sugar). Glucose is preferable to sucrose, because all of its effect occurs rapidly. As previously discussed, sucrose is a disaccharide consisting of a molecule of glucose bound to a molecule of fructose. It is digested rapidly and the glucose portion raises BG right away. The fructose portion must be first processed in the liver and will raise blood sugar later, when it is usually no longer low. Glucose is readily available in most packaged hard candies, which can be conveniently carried in a pocket. Packages of LIFESAVERS ®, and similar candies, usually list dextrose (glucose) or sugar (sucrose) as their principal ingredient and therefore are satisfactory for this purpose. Perhaps the most suitable commercial product for treatment of hypoglycemia is DEXTROSOL ®.[1] In this product, 14 flavored tablets are packed in a foil-wrapped, pocket-

1. Made by Brown and Polson Division, CPC United Kingdom, Ltd., Esher, Surrey KT 109 PN, England.

size package. Each tablet contains 2.8 grams of glucose and no sucrose, fructose, or oligosaccharides. The product thus will raise BG more rapidly than other candies, sugar cubes, or fruits and does *not* continue to raise BG for long periods after the initial action. The tablets dissolve rapidly in the mouth and do not become sticky in hot weather. DEXTROSOL is sold at candy and drug counters as a confection in Canada, England, Europe, and elsewhere. As an accommodation to users of this manual, DEXTROSOL is now available in the U.S. from Sugarfree Center for Diabetics, P.O. Box 114, Van Nuys, CA 91408. Five packages sell for $2.50 postpaid and substantial discounts are available on large orders.

How many little candies should be consumed for a given hypoglycemic episode? To know this, we must know the actual BG, the target BG, and the amount by which one candy raises BG. This last amount may differ from one patient to the next. For example, one DEXTROSOL will raise the BG of a Type Ia patient weighing 120–150 pounds by about 15 mg/dl. Thus if such a patient had a BG of 70 mg/dl and his target BG were 100 mg/dl, he would eat 2 DEXTROSOL tablets.[2]

Once treated, symptoms of hypoglycemia may persist even after BG has returned to the target value. This is because blood levels of catecholamines are high and take perhaps ½-hour to return to normal. It is the catecholamines that are responsible for the trembling, sweating, tachycardia (high pulse rate), and most other symptoms of hypoglycemia. Nevertheless, a patient who has treated his hypoglycemia in the fashion described can be assured that BG has been normalized. He should not succumb to the common temptation of eating until symptoms vanish. About ½-hour after treatment, another BG measurement should be made to ensure that BG has not started to drop again.

---

2. Or 3 LIFESAVERS ® @ 10 mg/dl, but they work a bit more slowly than DEXTROSOL.

Calibration of Sweets in BG Units

It is a relatively simple matter to calibrate any candy, glucose tablet, or sugar cube, or cherries, grapes, raisins, and other fruit, for the amount of BG increase that will be produced. The method, which follows, is very similar to the procedure, already discussed, for calibrating the effect of insulin on BG.

1. Measure BG. Proceed with experiment only if BG is at or below 100 mg/dl—so that it won't be raised too high.

2. Wait 15 minutes and measure BG again. It must be exactly the same as before, indicating that BG is holding steady. If BG has changed, the experiment will have to wait for an occasion when it remains constant.

3. Eat enough of the sweet product to provide about 6 grams of simple sugars. Examples of typical amounts would include:

DEXTROSOL, 2

Raisins, 1 tablespoon

Marshmallows (they don't stick in teeth when chewed), 2 standard-sized

Cherries, fresh (large), 6

Orange juice, ¼ cup

Sugar cubes, wrapped, 2

Grapes (large), 7

LIFESAVERS, fruit flavors, 3

These amounts will raise BG by about 30 mg/dl in many Type Ia adults but the calibration must be performed if precise results are to be obtained.

4. Measure BG ½-hour after step 3. Measure it again after 1 hour and then again after 1½ hours. Do not engage in strenuous physical activity during the measurement period, as this may affect the experiment. The maximum increase above the first BG is the value we are seeking.

5. Once you have obtained the maximum increase, per-

form a simple division to calculate the effect of the quantity
consumed on BG, as in the following examples:

	mg/dl
Final BG	120
Minus initial BG	− 90
BG increase	30

30 mg/dl ÷ 3 LIFESAVERS = 10 mg/dl per LIFESAVER

	mg/dl
Final BG	135
Minus initial BG	−100
BG increase	35

35 mg/dl ÷ 7 grapes = 5 mg/dl per grape

Calibration of sweets should be entered on the GLUCO-
GRAF Data Sheet. If the calibrations change, the new ones
should be entered. Entries should be recopied onto the next
Data Sheet so that they are not forgotten. If a product takes
longer than ½ hour to exert 90 percent of its BG effect, it is
unsuitable for treatment of hypoglycemia (except when
nothing else is on hand).

Avoiding BG "Overshoot," or Rebound, When Treating Hypoglycemia

For many years, it was believed that hypoglycemic BG
levels frequently initiated an overwhelming release of counter-regulatory hormones, which would raise BG to very high
levels (hyperglycemia). This supposed response is commonly
called the Somogyi effect, perpetuating the name of the in-
vestigator who proposed it more than 20 years ago. Our experience with frequent BG monitoring by a number of
patients over a period of six years indicates that *the most*

common cause of BG rebound after hypoglycemia is the administration of too much food or the wrong kind of food. (A group of investigators in Nottingham, England, recently confirmed another form of BG rebound. It will occur when blood insulin levels are initially too high [causing hypoglycemia] but are subsequently too low. This happens, for example, in patients taking one daily injection of NPH or Lente insulin. In such cases, high blood insulin levels appear 8 hours after injection, but drop to negligible levels after, perhaps, 13 hours. Thus BG went down after 8 hours, and then up, several hours later.)

The extreme range of daily BG levels in Type Ia patients is usually due to the following sequence of events:

1. High insulin dose to cover high-carbohydrate diet.

2. At certain times of the day, blood insulin levels are too high (these peaks do not usually occur with the low doses of long-acting insulin that we advocate).

3. Patient eats too much *or* the wrong kind of food in an attempt to reverse the resulting hypoglycemia.

4. BG increases to hyperglycemic levels.

5. Patient takes Regular insulin to correct the high BG, but guesses incorrectly at the amount to administer.

6. BG drops too far and the cycle goes on and on, like an endless roller coaster.

Type Ib diabetics (producing a fair amount of endogenous insulin) are subject to a further problem. If they eat a meal shortly after a hypoglycemic episode, their insulin response to that meal will be reduced, even if BG has been normalized. As a result they can expect an elevated BG after a meal that would ordinarily cause no problems.

What is the wrong kind of food for reversing hypoglycemia? Any food that takes more than ½ hour to *complete* its effect upon BG should not be used for this purpose. The patient clearly needs something that works within a few minutes, and then stops. The antiquated treatments of milk and crackers, cheese, and other foods that are high in protein, fat, or complex carbohydrates will exert most of their BG effect after ½ hour, when BG elevation is not desired, rather than within 10 minutes, when it is urgently needed. Many diabetics use hypoglycemia as an occasion for eating their favorite forbidden or restricted foods. Common examples of such inappropriate delicacies are peanut butter, ice cream, yogurt, and pastries, which usually contain some simple sugars but principally consist of polysaccharides or fats.

Proteins and fats, if eaten before or with simple sugars or other carbohydrates, can actually slow BG rise. Thus 10 grams of pure sucrose will raise BG much more rapidly if the stomach is empty than if some cheese or milk were eaten first. (This knowledge can be of help to patients who are late or early for a planned meal. If late, but not known to be hypoglycemic, eat the carbohydrate portion of the meal before the protein or fat portions. If early, and therefore fearful of raising BG before enough injected insulin has reached the bloodstream, eat the protein and fat portions [meat, etc.] of the meal, before eating the carbohydrate portions [vegetables, bread, etc.]. If the early meal includes a salad containing only vegetables with mostly nonabsorbable carbohydrate [see page 161], then that should also be eaten first.)

Now that we have eliminated from consideration the inappropriate foods for reversing hypoglycemia, we are back to the simple sugars. Ideal sources that are convenient to carry and to calibrate are packaged hard candies and cubes of table sugar. DEXTROSOL, mentioned previously, is especially useful and fast-acting. Many patients prefer to calibrate fruits, because they feel that fruits are "natural" foods and that candies are somehow "harmful" to diabetics. This thinking is particularly absurd when it comes to the treatment of hypoglycemia, where prompt effect, without "overshoot," should be the prime consideration. Most chewable hard candies will serve this purpose very well. Table sugar will give a fast response from the glucose half and then a slower response from the fructose. Some fruits contain high levels of fructose and much lower amounts of glucose. Therefore if fruits are to be used for treating hypoglycemia, their effect should be checked by BG monitoring, to make sure that most of the rise occurs within the first ½ hour. Such speedy action from fruits is unusual and we therefore do not recommend fruit for this purpose.

Some patients prefer to carry plastic tubes of a glucose solution such as GLUTOSE ® [3] or INSTANT GLUCOSE.[4] These are excellent for administration to a confused or semi-conscious person, but pose some problems for routine self-treatment:

1. Inconvenient to carry in pocket.

2. Contains about triple the amount of glucose needed for a typical insulin reaction.

3. Difficult to calibrate because the plastic bottle has no volumetric markings.

4. Tube can leak if closed after use.

Liquids (including liquid glucose) should not be administered to an unconscious person (who can choke). Glucagon should be injected.

We can now conclude that the ideal procedure for self-treatment of hypoglycemia is as follows:

1. Carry, at all times, a package of hard candies (preferably DEXTROSOL), with glucose or dextrose listed on the label, as principal (first) ingredient. These should have been previously calibrated for their effect on BG.

2. At first suspicion of hypoglycemia, measure BG.

---

3. Paddock Laboratories, Inc., 2744 Lyndale Avenue, South Minneapolis, Minn. 55408.

4. Diabetes Assoc. of Greater Cleveland, 2022 Lee Road, Cleveland, Ohio 44118.

3. Immediately, eat enough calibrated candies to bring BG up to target value (usually 100 mg/dl).

4. WAIT for candies to take effect. Do not rush to take additional candies if symptoms persist.

5. Measure BG again after ½ hour, and then, if necessary, take additional candies.

6. If without reagent strips, and resting pulse is rapid, assume that the symptoms truly reflect hypoglycemia and eat enough candies to raise BG by 70–80 mg/dl. For most Type Ia adults, this will be about 7 LIFESAVERS or 5 DEXTROSOL. This should be adequate for treating a BG of zero.

7. Some hypoglycemic episodes, and certainly the use of glucagon, will totally deplete the glycogen stored in the liver. This may increase the hazard of subsequent hypoglycemia later in the day, so measure BG frequently, during the balance of the day, to catch low BG before it becomes too severe.

8. Record details of any hypoglycemic episodes on the data sheet, including BG before and after sweets, as well as the number of sweets consumed. This data will serve as an important check on the validity of the original calibration of the sweets.

Treatment When Hypoglycemia Results in the Patient Becoming Confused or Semiconscious

This is an emergency situation, in which BG rebound is no longer a significant consideration. Family, close friends, and fellow employees, or fellow students, teachers, and other associates should be advised, in advance, of the appropriate procedure and of the likelihood that the patient may resist treatment.

Ideally, the patient will have in a pocket, purse, or desk a plastic squeeze bottle of liquid glucose (page 187). The glucose should be slowly squirted into the mouth—in the space between the cheeks and the teeth, to minimize danger of choking. One-half bottle of glucose solution should be adequate (one bottle of GLUTOSE contains 32 grams of glucose). If the patient is uncooperative (very common), don't be put off. Insist that he drink.

If the patient is lucid enough to drink without assistance, instead of the glucose solution he can be given any of the following:

1. Glass of warm water with 5 packets or cubes of table sugar dissolved in it.

2. Two glasses of orange juice or soft drink, or one glass containing three packets of dissolved sugar. Low-calorie or dietary soft drinks are worthless unless fortified with packets of sugar.

When the patient becomes rational, he should immediately measure BG and take calibrated sweets, if necessary. He should check BG again after ½ hour and correct any deviation from target value with sweets (if low BG), or Regular insulin (if high BG). BG measurements every 1–2 hours will be warranted because of the glycogen depletion mentioned in the preceding section.

Treating Hypoglycemia in the Unconscious Patient

Again, family, friends, fellow employees, and other close associates should be taught the following procedures:

The ideal treatment is the prompt injection, subcutaneously (like insulin) of glucagon (available from Eli Lilly & Co., Indianapolis, Ind. 46206). Lilly currently supplies glucagon in a box containing instructions for use and two tiny glass vials. A small plastic carrying case is available on special request. One vial contains powdered glucagon and the other contains 1 cc of distilled water. The two are mixed, according to instructions, and injected. Any 1-cc insulin syringe may be used. If only ½-cc syringes are on hand, use only half the water, mixed with *all* of the powder. The entire mixed solution should be injected. Although an overdose is not possible, a half-dose is preferred for small children and a double dose (2 vials of powder) for large adults. Since this dose of glucagon will convert to blood glucose all glycogen stored in the liver, there is a real danger of lessened glycogen protection from subsequent drops of BG. It is therefore especially necessary for the patient to measure BG frequently during the next 24 hours. Careful maintenance of *normal* (not high) BG, for one day, will insure the restoration of adequate glycogen reserves, provided the usual meals are eaten.

If major changes that may affect BG control are occurring (for example, pregnancy, new insulin or diet regimen, serious illness), play it safe. Prefill a syringe with glucagon and tape it to a wall, side of desk, or other convenient location, and show it to relatives or associates. Tell them how and when to use it. Do not try to go through major changes in isolation.

If the glucagon is not available, neither fluids nor solid sweets should be placed in the mouth of the unconscious patient, since these can cause choking. Instead, the patient should be immediately hospitalized. In fact, it is proper to summon an ambulance even after administration of glucagon, if the patient does not regain consciousness within 3 minutes. Ambulance crews are frequently equipped to inject 50 percent dextrose (glucose) solution intravenously, a treatment that instantly raises BG. (15 cc of 50 percent dextrose will raise BG from zero to about 115 mg/dl in an average adult.)

When a hypoglycemic patient is unconscious, there is a good likelihood that convulsions may occur. During convulsions, the tightly clamped teeth can bite into the tongue, causing serious damage. This can be prevented by placing a rolled-up handkerchief between the rear teeth on one side of the mouth. The handkerchief should not protrude so far into the mouth that it will block the airway.

After recovery from any episode of hypoglycemia, efforts should be made to determine its cause.

Hypoglycemia After a Meal

The patient should try to recall if the episode was precipitated by too long a time interval between a preprandial dose of R and eating the meal. If so, he should not bring BG all the way back to the target value, because digestion of the meal will eventually take care of that. Instead, it may be wise to settle for a BG about 15 percent below target. This procedure can prevent a subsequent BG rise to abnormal levels.

Impaired Sexual Functioning When Blood Glucose Is Low

Many insulin-dependent diabetics who monitor BG have discovered that inability to become aroused, or, if aroused, inability to achieve orgasm, can be early warnings of hypoglycemia. Naturally, this is not the only cause of sexual dysfunction but for insulin users it's probably the most common. This early warning sign has been detected by both males and females. In fact, some patients have located the BG's at which they "turn off."

It appears that both men and women tend to have two turn-off points—at a certain BG they can be aroused but cannot achieve orgasm. At a lower BG they cannot even be aroused. Furthermore, many men awake nearly every morning with a penile erection (a natural occurrence during a certain stage of sleep) and find that failure to do so is frequently an indicator of low BG. Some patients try to prevent an unpleasant situation by measuring BG (when feasible) prior to anticipated intercourse and promptly taking fast-acting sweets if BG is low.

We have discussed the subject of hypoglycemia in more detail than one usually encounters because very few texts deal adequately with this urgent subject. We do not expect patients on our regimen to become unconscious. In fact, we anticipate considerable relief from the high frequency of hypoglycemic episodes usually encountered in patients who take large doses of intermediate- or long-acting insulin. Nevertheless, it is sensible to be properly prepared.

15

EXERCISE AND BLOOD GLUCOSE
CONTROL

SUMMARY

Diabetics who engage in a moderate level of daily activity appear to be easier to control than those who are sedentary. It has been a long-held myth, however, that *strenuous* or endurance exercise facilitates BG control. While such exercise can relieve emotional stress and may also reduce cardiovascular risk, it usually introduces major complexities in attempts to control insulin-dependent diabetes. Nevertheless, we heartily recommend regular exercise and try in this chapter to present a method for circumventing some of the problems it poses for BG control. Topics covered include:

1. Intense or prolonged exercise—benefits and problems.
2. Biochemistry of glucose utilization by muscle.
3. The effects of exercise upon blood glucose level.
4. How to maintain normal BG during and after the first exercise session.
5. Analyzing the data from the first exercise period.
6. How to maintain normal BG during and after subsequent typical exercise sessions.

Intense or Prolonged Exercise—Benefits and Problems

Many diabetics who engage in regular athletic activities feel that their physical and, perhaps, emotional well-being owe much to their sports participation. Many physicians subscribe to the notion that strenuous or endurance exercise somehow facilitates control of BG, yet there is no evidence in the scientific literature to support this viewpoint. Regular exercise can lower insulin requirements but this is not synonymous with improved control (more constant BG's which are nearer to normal). Clinical experience indicates, however, that sedentary patients are more difficult to control than patients who get a moderate daily level of physical activity, whether in their jobs or by participation in sports.

It is suspected (but not proved) that nondiabetics who exercise, either moderately or strenuously, are less subject to the various blood vessel (vascular) and heart (cardiac) diseases that affect our aging population. From time to time references appear in the popular press, describing diabetic athletes who, while not putting special care into control of BG, manage to survive many years, without the major complications of their disease. If this really turns out to be true, current theory provides no certain explanation for the phenomenon. It has been shown, however, that nondiabetic individuals, placed on strenuous exercise regimens, experience marked improvement of serum cholesterol, triglyceride, and HDL values (see Chapter 7) as well as significant reductions in heart rate and systolic blood pressure at rest and during submaximal work. These people also exhibit an increased fibrinolytic activity (ability of blood to dissolve small clots) in response to experimental blockage of blood vessels. Since all these values deteriorate in poorly controlled diabetes and may be relevant to the high incidence of cardiac and vascular disease among diabetics, this point may be very important to the long-term goals of therapy.

On the other hand, patients on the GLUCOGRAF regimen are usually very well controlled and generally experience reasonably normal blood values for the aforementioned lipids. Unless considerable care is taken, strenuous exercise programs introduce a factor that can make proper control of BG very difficult. This chapter considers the means by which a patient can engage in strenuous exercise without seriously disturbing BG control.

During exercise, blood flow is diverted from the kidneys to the muscles and therefore exercise programs may be inappropriate for some diabetics with pre-existing kidney disease. While exercising, blood pressure usually increases, thereby enhancing the danger of retinal hemorrhage in patients with certain forms of retinopathy.

Biochemistry of Glucose Utilization by Muscle

In resting or slowly exercising muscle, the energy contained in the chemical bonds that hold a glucose or a fatty acid (derived from fat) molecule together is gradually transferred, by a process called oxidation, to a molecule called ATP (adenosine triphosate) that contains two bonds of very high energy. The energy of one of these bonds can be released very rapidly and is used directly by muscle filaments to move little ratchets on their surfaces that cause the filaments to slide against one another and thereby perform work.

Oxidation is a relatively slow process entailing many biochemical steps and relying upon the transport of 12 atoms of oxygen for every glucose molecule that is oxidized. Oxygen molecules must first be inhaled with air, transferred to capillary blood vessels in the lungs, attached to hemoglobin in red blood cells, released from the bloodstream when they reach muscle, and transferred across the outer membrane of muscle cells. Finally the oxygen molecules are carried inside the

muscle cell to a special structure in the cell called the mito-
chondrion where they finally pick up electrons generated
during the total breakdown of glucose (or fatty acid) to car-
bon dioxide. As the oxygen acquires the electrons, it associates with hydrogen to form water.

Oxidation is a very efficient process in that one glucose
molecule can produce high energy bonds for about 36 molecules of ATP. Slowly exercising muscle therefore utilizes relatively little glucose in comparison to the amount of oxygen
used. In contrast, resting muscle relies almost exclusively on
the oxidation of fatty acids for energy, so virtually no glucose
is utilized.

During exercise, respiration and heart rates increase to
meet the oxygen needs of the activity. When the rate of
muscle activity finally exceeds the rate at which oxygen can
be transported to the mitochondria, another process takes
over for extracting energy from glucose. This process, called
anaerobic (without air or oxygen) glycolysis (splitting of
glucose), requires no oxygen. It does not break down glucose
completely but splits it in half to form 2 molecules of lactic
acid. Because the full energy of the glucose molecule is not
extracted, bond energy is transferred to only 2 ATP molecules. Strenuous activity or anaerobic glycolysis cannot be
sustained for extended periods because the lactic acid accumulates faster than it can be removed and muscle ceases to
function at the resulting high acid levels.

Since, from 1 molecule of glucose, aerobic oxidation provides high energy bonds for about 36 ATP molecules,
whereas anaerobic glycolysis can produce bonds for only 2
ATP molecules, it is evident that for the same amount of
muscular work, about 18 times as much glucose is needed for
anaerobic glycolysis as for aerobic oxidation.

In practice, one rarely exercises a given muscle entirely

aerobically or entirely anaerobically. Usually high-intensity exercise that can only be tolerated for short periods involves more anaerobic muscle cells and uses up blood glucose very rapidly. Steady-state exercise that can be continued for long periods is principally aerobic and uses blood glucose very slowly.

By way of examples—a high-intensity workout on a stationary exercise bicycle set for high resistance might be mostly anaerobic. A 50-mile bicycle race, although very tiring, would probably entail mostly aerobic activity. Aerobic activity in muscle tends to predominate when heart rate is less than 85 percent of an individual's maximum possible rate. Above this point exercise may be called "strenuous." Because it can sometimes be dangerous for a person to exercise at maximum heart rate, a rule of thumb has been developed that is utilized by exercise physiologists when working with untrained people: "Maximum heart rate is approximately 220 beats per minute minus the age in years." Thus an untrained 30-year-old would typically have a maximum heart rate of about $220 - 30 = 190$ beats per minute. Strenuous exercise for this person would theoretically be that which produces a heart rate equal to or greater than 85 percent $\times$ 190 $=$ 162 beats per minute.[1] A simple but crude indicator that someone is exercising in the anaerobic range is inability to converse comfortably.

It is interesting to note that the muscles of trained athletes can utilize fatty acids for a substantial portion of their energy requirements. They may therefore use up less glucose for a given amount of work than people who are untrained. This is important because it implies that a well-trained diabetic athlete may experience less disturbance of BG for a given workout than will a diabetic who is not "in shape."

---

1. See pages 180–181 for suggestions on measuring pulse (heart) rate.

The Effects of Exercise upon Blood Glucose Level

Strenuous exercise can, for diabetics, affect BG by a number of independent mechanisms, some of which may occur simultaneously and some of which may only occur rarely in a particular patient:

1. If any type of insulin is injected in a site over a muscle that will be exercised, the subsequent exercise can triple the rate of release of this insulin into the bloodstream. This is, perhaps, the principal cause of severe hypoglycemia during and after strenuous exercise. The rapid release of such insulin will make it unavailable later, when it may be needed. It is, therefore, wise to decide the nature of exercise before administering insulin and then to inject in a region of the body that will not be exercised. Thus an individual who plans to run or jog should inject the preceding doses of insulin into the arm or abdomen, rather than into the thigh. This phenomenon can be put to good use if a patient has a high BG that he wishes to lower very rapidly. He can, for example, inject Regular insulin, subcutaneously, into the thigh and then pedal his exercise bicycle rapidly for 15 minutes. Alternately he can inject into an arm and then do push-ups, chins, and other exercises of the upper arm. It should be possible to push most of the Regular insulin into the bloodstream in 1 hour instead of 2–3 hours.

2. Exercising muscle utilizes glucose as an energy source much more rapidly than resting muscle (which principally utilizes fatty acids), provided that there is a high enough blood level of insulin to facilitate entry of glucose into muscle cells. Aerobic exercise utilizes glucose very efficiently, so that relatively little glucose will supply enough energy for a considerable amount of work. Aerobic or mild exercise can lower BG in diabetics who have adequate blood levels of insulin, but it will not lower BG very rapidly. If aerobic

exercise is continued for extended periods, hypoglycemia can be produced.

3. During strenuous or anaerobic exercise, glucose is consumed at a very high rate. It would take about 18 grams of glucose to provide as many calories to the same muscle exercising anaerobically as 1 gram can provide to an aerobically exercising muscle. We can therefore conclude that prolonged intermittent anaerobic exercise will rapidly lower BG in insulin-treated diabetics. During 40-minute periods containing numerous spurts of anaerobic exercise,[2] the author has experienced BG reductions (continually countered with glucose tablets) of 200 mg/dl, for an average BG reduction of 5 mg/dl per minute. Because of the pain involved (due to accumulation of lactic acid and bradykinin in muscles), anaerobic exercise is difficult to endure and is not commonly practiced, except by body builders and very serious competitive athletes. The borderline of muscular activity that involves simultaneous aerobic and anaerobic metabolism is probably ideal for building strength, stamina, and muscle mass, but is hard to define. Training at this level, by middle-aged individuals and by patients with any diabetic complications, should be approached gradually and only upon the advice of a knowledgeable physician. Any level of exercise that substantially increases blood pressure can cause hemorrhaging in sighted diabetics with certain forms of clinically discernible retinopathy such as microaneurisms.

4. Upon the onset of exercise, several hormonal counter-regulatory systems become active, making additional blood glucose available for muscular consumption. This occurs in both diabetics and nondiabetics and includes increased blood levels of catecholamines, glucocorticoids, growth hormone, and glucagon. In the nondiabetic, insulin release slows down. If exercise is terminated shortly after starting, before the

---

2. Anaerobic exercise cannot be maintained continuously for more than a few minutes at a time.

newly released glucose has been fully utilized, BG levels will be elevated. In the nondiabetic, this is countered by an increase in insulin release so that BG is rapidly normalized. But the insulin-dependent diabetic is slowly releasing injected long-acting insulin at a rate that can be neither speeded up nor slowed by BG level. A brief spurt of exercise for him can actually cause an increase of BG that will not be offset by release of more insulin. This leaves us with a simple lesson—a diabetic wanting to lower BG should run for a bus only if the bus stop is at least ½ mile away, because a brief dash is more likely to raise BG than to lower it.

5. Can exercise substitute for insulin as a means of lowering BG? Sometimes it can, and sometimes it will actually cause BG to rise. When BG is low, normal, or slightly elevated, perhaps as high as 150 mg/dl, strenuous exercise will usually cause BG to drop. At such levels, when BG is not too far above normal, there is usually enough circulating insulin to facilitate muscular uptake of glucose. When BG is in the vicinity of perhaps 200 mg/dl and above, the patient is usually in a state of relative insulinopenia (too little insulin in the blood). His muscles will utilize energy from body fats, rather than from glucose—which cannot enter muscle cells in the absence of insulin. Furthermore, as indicated in the preceding paragraph, counter-regulatory hormones are entering the circulation. In this instance, they may not be opposed by significant amounts of insulin. This relative lack of insulin can lead to an eightfold increase in exercise-induced blood levels of catecholamines. The liver then breaks down proteins and glycogen, producing more glucose. Fats may also be broken down for energy and ketones will be released as a by-product. Thus, the substitution of exercise for insulin, when BG is over perhaps 200 mg/dl (and for some people, over 150 mg/dl), can lead to both higher BG and ketosis

(ketones in the blood). The BG values at which these problems may occur will vary from one person to another and will depend upon many other factors including blood insulin level.

6. Exercise appears to produce an increased tissue sensitivity to insulin that can last 24 hours or more beyond the actual exercise period. This is especially noticeable when exercise has been of high intensity or prolonged. When muscles are exercised strenuously, first some muscle proteins break down and then additional muscle tissue is built. The breakdown process produces elevated blood levels of small polypeptides (protein fractions) called kinins. It is believed, by some investigators, that these kinins enhance the effectiveness of insulin. Other investigators observe that the number of high-affinity insulin receptors in body tissues increases after exercise. Furthermore, since muscle and liver glycogen are depleted during strenuous or prolonged exercise, these stores must be rebuilt during the next 24 hours. The process of rebuilding glycogen (glycogenesis) will consume blood glucose and thereby lower BG. The rebuilding of muscle tissue requires protein building blocks (amino acids) and a source of energy—usually derived from glucose. The sum of all these effects, taken together, can bring about a fair reduction in need for long-acting insulin in patients who exercise daily or even every other day. When regular exercise is pursued for a period of several months, the reduced need for insulin may continue for as long as two weeks after cessation of exercise. Whatever the cause, the net result can be periods of hypoglycemia, throughout the day, especially during the 3 hours after exercising.

This can be avoided by reducing all daily doses of long-acting insulin and by following the procedure set forth in the next section.

How to Maintain Normal BG During and After the First Exercise Session

The following procedure is an approximate guide. It should be modified to conform to the patient's target BG and measured responses to sweets and insulin. *An exercise program should not be embarked upon until BG has been stabilized with diet and insulin. Premature addition of exercise to the regimen will make control more difficult.*

1. Measure BG immediately before exercising. If it is in the 130–150 mg/dl range, take no immediate corrective measures.

2. If BG is greater than 150 mg/dl, take enough Regular insulin to bring it down to 130 mg/dl. Inject in a site that overlies the muscles to be exercised. Do not exercise until BG drops below 200 mg/dl.

3. If BG is below 100 mg/dl, eat enough calibrated candies or glucose tablets to bring it up to 100 mg/dl. Wait until this BG level has been attained before starting to exercise.

4. If BG is in the range of 100–130 mg/dl, eat a source of simple sugars or oligosaccharides that has been calibrated to raise BG by 15–20 mg/dl. This can be candy, or small fruit, such as cherries, grapes, or raisins. Immediately begin to exercise.

5. During the first exercise period, measure BG every 10 or 15 minutes or every 2 miles (for example) if running, etc. Certainly measure BG at the first sign of hypoglycemia.

6. After each BG measurement, eat enough calibrated sweets to bring BG up to 100 mg/dl and to anticipate the next drop in BG. Stop exercising temporarily if BG drops below 70 mg/dl or if valid hypoglycemic symptoms appear. Thus, for example, suppose that initial BG was 100 mg/dl,

and one candy, good for 15 mg/dl, was eaten before exercising. Fifteen minutes later, BG is 85 mg/dl. Then the exercise would have caused a BG drop of 15 + 15 = 30 mg/dl, if the candy had not been eaten. Therefore, after the 85 mg/dl measurement, eat three 15 mg/dl candies and continue exercising. By the end of the next 15 minutes, BG should be almost exactly 100 mg/dl. (BG would have fallen 30 mg/dl, from 85 to 55, without candy; 3 candies [45 mg/dl] would bring it up to 100.)

7. Continue to exercise, to measure BG, and to eat calibrated sweets, if necessary, every 10–15 minutes or every 2 miles, etc. Keep a written record of time (or miles), BG values, and number of sweets eaten.

8. Upon concluding the first exercise period, again measure and record BG and, if needed, eat additional sweets to bring BG up to 100 mg/dl. If BG is elevated, but below 150 mg/dl, do not take any insulin, since BG will probably drop to within the target range if exercise has been strenuous or prolonged. If BG is greater than 150 mg/dl, take enough Regular insulin to bring it to the upper limit of target range.

9. After exercise, measure BG every hour for the next 3 hours. This is to ascertain any hypoglycemia before symptoms occur.

10. Be sure to enter on the Data Sheet all measurements and all sweets taken.

Analyzing the Data from the First Exercise Period

The preceding steps should have been performed before, during, and after the first exercise period. This was a trial to get an approximate idea of the effects of a particular form of exercise on a particular patient. We must now utilize that data, in order to simplify our efforts in controlling BG at subsequent exercise sessions.

Consider the following data, gathered by a hypothetical patient during the first exercise session:

8:00 P.M.   BG 80, 2 DEXTROSOL (each worth 15 mg/dl). Will start exercising when BG exceeds 100 mg/dl.
8:25   BG 110, 1 DEXTROSOL, started exercise on stationary bicycle.
8:40   BG 95, 2 DEXTROSOL, continued exercise.
8:55   BG 92, 2 DEXTROSOL, continued exercise.
9:10   BG 88, end of exercise, 1 DEXTROSOL.
10:10   BG 58, 3 DEXTROSOL.
11:10   BG 105.
12:10   BG 105.

Now let us analyze the data:

BG at start of exercise	(8:25)	110 mg/dl
Minus BG at end of exercise	(9:10)	88 mg/dl
Net drop in BG during exercise		22 mg/dl

DEXTROSOL consumed:

8:25 P.M.	1 tablet, started exercise
8:40	2 tablets, during exercise
8:55	2 tablets, during exercise
	Total 5 tablets

Note that the total does not include the first 2 tablets taken at 8:00 P.M. They served only to bring BG up to starting point and not to offset the effects of exercise. Nor was the tablet taken when exercise stopped, at 9:10, counted because its effect on BG occurred after the 9:10 measurement.

Thus, in spite of consuming 5 tablets @ 15 mg/dl, BG dropped by 22 mg/dl after 45 minutes of exercise. This is equivalent to a total BG drop of (5 tablets × 15 mg/dl) + 22 mg/dl = 75 + 22 = 97 mg/dl, over a 45-minute period. Therefore, for this patient and this type of exercise, BG will drop 97 mg/dl in 45 minutes = 2 mg/dl per minute, while exercising. Therefore, every 7 minutes BG will drop about 14 mg/dl, or the approximate value of 1 DEXTROSOL tablet. Thus if this patient exercises on the stationary bike again the next day, he should start off with a BG in the upper half of his target range, he should eat 1 DEXTROSOL tablet as he begins, and he should eat 1 additional tablet every 7 minutes until he stops.

Now, the original data shows that BG continued to drop for 1 hour after exercising. It dropped from 88 mg/dl at 9:10 to 58 mg/dl at 10:10, in spite of eating a DEXTROSOL at 9:10 worth 15 mg/dl. Therefore the effective drop during the first hour after exercise was $(88 - 58) + (1 \times 15) = 30 + 15 = 45$ mg/dl. This could have been covered by a total of 3 DEXTROSOL tablets taken as follows:

1 tablet upon termination of exercise.

1 tablet 20 minutes after termination of exercise.

1 tablet 40 minutes after termination of exercise.

Since BG no longer dropped after the first hour, it is likely that if the next day the patient takes 1 tablet every 7 minutes while exercising and then 3 tablets over the next 40 minutes, he will maintain his starting BG level continuously.

This example leads to the following program for BG maintenance, during subsequent exercise sessions:

How to Maintain Normal BG During and After Subsequent Typical Exercise Sessions

1. Know the BG calibration of the sweets that will be used. Note that small fruits may be acceptable for *preventing* hypoglycemia but may be too slow to act in *treating* hypoglycemia, once it begins. If exercise is to be prolonged for more than 1½ hours, it may even be practical to prevent hypoglycemia by using slower-acting CHO, such as cookies or milk, at the start of the exercise period, instead of small amounts of quick-acting CHO throughout the exercise period.

2. Know how many minutes (or miles, etc.) of exercise at a given heart rate [3] can be covered by 1 sweet.

3. Start exercising when BG is in the upper half of the target range. BG must be measured.

4. Eat 1 sweet when starting. Eat additional sweets according to the calibration of paragraph number 2, this section (for example, every 10 minutes).

5. Measure BG when exercise is half-finished, as a double check that it is responding as planned. Correct with sweets, if BG is low, and do not continue exercise until BG reaches target range. If BG has increased above normal, hold back the appropriate number of sweets when continuing to exercise.

6. Measure BG at termination of exercise and use sweets to raise BG, if necessary. If BG is higher than target range, but within, perhaps, 30 mg/dl of the top of that range, do not correct with insulin.

7. During the post-exercise period, eat additional sweets, spaced appropriately in time, if this was indicated by the data taken on the first day.

8. Measure BG, during or after exercise, whenever there is any suspicion of hypoglycemia.

9. Continue any regularly scheduled preprandial and postprandial BG measurements.

10. Record all BG measurements, exercise type, and intensity (for example, heart rate), time spent,[4] and sweets consumed. Use this information to revise the procedure for covering exercise, until BG remains within target range during and after all exercise sessions.

Are three BG measurements for every exercise session really worth the trouble? Consider the time and effort de-

---

3. See pages 180–181 for suggestions on measuring pulse (heart) rate.

4. This information is also of value for checking progress in building endurance during a cardiorespiratory training program, where the goal is progressively to increase exercise intensity without increasing heart rate.

voted to these measurements—perhaps 5 minutes. Now consider the time and effort put into exercising, including clothing change, shower, and so forth. Also consider the time that may be wasted if unnecessary hypoglycemia occurs, and the weariness that usually follows hypoglycemia. It appears that a bargain return is received on a small investment of time.

Once an exercise program is in effect, watch out for unexpected hypoglycemia at times unrelated to the periods of exercise. This is a sign that regular exercise has lowered the necessary dose of long- (or intermediate-) acting insulin. If the hypoglycemia occurs several days in succession, lower each dose of long-acting insulin by ½ unit. If hypoglycemia is severe (BG below 50 mg/dl) or recurs during the day, lower each dose by 1 unit. Further reductions should be made if hypoglycemia continues, but remember that UL keeps acting for up to 4 days, so try to wait 3 days between dosage changes.

Also learn to distinguish fatigue from hypoglycemia. Inability to work out at a customary level of intensity can be due to either cause. Check BG to be certain. Terminate exercise, at least temporarily, when BG is below the target range—not only because of the potential hazard, but also because exercising when BG is low will not build strength or endurance and can be very exhausting.

16

BLOOD GLUCOSE CONTROL DURING
ILLNESS OR INFECTION

SUMMARY

Ketoacidosis, which may be precipitated by illness or infection, is a frequent cause of hospitalization in IDDM. With the tools and knowledge we now have, this condition is totally avoidable with relatively little effort. The brevity of this chapter attests to the simplicity with which a heretofore very difficult situation can be handled today. Topics covered include:

1. BG control when diet is unchanged.
2. BG control when diet has been reduced or patient is not eating.
3. Ketosis and ketoacidosis.
4. Oral medications containing sugars.

Although a patient may be fully capable of controlling BG on his own, it is essential that the physician be promptly and continuously consulted throughout the course of any illness that affects BG control. This is usually a situation in which the added experience of a professional becomes very important.

Most diabetics, especially those requiring exogenous insulin, frequently experience increased difficulty controlling

BG in cases of systemic viral or bacterial infections (colds, pneumonia, intestinal virus, flu, mumps, measles, etc.). Less frequent, although not uncommon, is a similar response in the presence of local infections, such as those brought on by traumatic injuries, dental surgery, etc. Illness and infection are associated with a marked reduction in the number of insulin receptors in both diabetics and nondiabetics. The consequence for IDDM is that the prior daily insulin dosage is no longer adequate and more insulin is needed. The reason for this strange response is not known. The net effect upon BG can sometimes be very considerable. In fact, infection ranks second only to omission of insulin dose as a predisposing factor for diabetic ketoacidosis.

Patients on our regimen observe that illness or infection usually appears to affect only their basal insulin requirement and not the insulin needed to cover meals (if the meals remain unchanged). That is, if they raise their long-acting or intermediate-acting dose, they can usually control BG without changing the doses of Regular insulin required for meals. Changes in dose of long-acting insulin can pose certain problems, which are discussed later in this chapter. It is therefore important that a patient be in telephone contact with his physician during periods of illness, and especially before experimenting with the dosage of long-acting insulin.

During illness, one of two possible situations usually occurs.

1. The patient is sick, but eating in accord with his usual diet.

2. The sick patient is eating less than his usual diet or is abstaining from food altogether.

The insulin regimens for these two situations are quite different. The two aspects of treatment that both situations may have in common are continuation of insulin therapy (with possible modification) and increased frequency of BG measurement.

BG Control When Diet Is Unchanged

1. When illness or infection occurs, do not increase any long-acting insulin dose, until the need for additional insulin has been clearly demonstrated by repeated measurement of BG. If a patient is routinely measuring BG with the frequency suggested on pages 92–93, he may even observe increased need for insulin before becoming aware of any illness. This may be the very first sign of illness.

What is a clearly demonstrated need for additional insulin? Perhaps the following typical example, translated from the Data Sheet of a hypothetical patient, will illustrate.

11:00 P.M.   BG 98, bedtime.
 7:00 A.M.   BG 150, usual morning insulin dose plus an extra 2R to lower elevated BG.
 8:45 A.M.   Breakfast, delayed 45 minutes longer than usual, to give BG a chance to drop.
11:00 A.M.   BG 170, 2½R to bring down BG.
 1:00 P.M.   BG 130; 11:00 A.M. dose has started to take effect. 5R, usual pre-lunch dose.
 2:00 P.M.   Lunch.
 4:30 P.M.   BG 140, 1R to bring down BG.

The day is less than half over and this patient has already required 2 + 2½ + 1 = 5½ units of additional Regular insulin over and above his usual dose. If this continues until the following morning, there will be a clear need for additional long-acting (or intermediate-acting) insulin.

2. In consultation with the physician, a plan should be made for temporarily increasing the dose of long- or intermediate-acting insulin. At first, the amount of increase should be limited to ½ the total extra units of Regular insulin injected in the prior 24 hours. Thus, if our hypothetical patient finished his day, having taken 8 units additional Regular insulin, he would increase his total dose of long- or intermediate-acting insulin by 8 ÷ 2 = 4 units, the next day. This

increase must be split, however, between his A.M. and P.M. doses. Thus, he would take 2 units extra in the morning and another 2 extra units in the evening.

This poses a problem if the patient is on Ultralente insulin. A dosage change in this insulin must usually be continued for 3 successive days before its full cumulative effect appears. Therefore the patient will not get the full benefit of the extra insulin until 3 days have elapsed. By that time, the illness may no longer be present, and the added insulin can cause hypoglycemia. There is a way of circumventing this problem, however:

a. If the patient is using Ultralente insulin, the additional insulin can be given as Lente insulin in 2 separate injections spaced exactly 12 hours apart. The Lente should probably not be mixed with the Ultralente, as it will change the activity curve of the Ultralente and thereby introduce another variable, whose effects may be difficult to predict. (Nevertheless, some physicians may wish to experiment with such mixtures.) The patient will thus be receiving at least 5 daily injections while ill. By this time, he is so used to multiple daily doses, that the two additional injections are probably of little significance. If Lente is mixed with Ultralente, the Regular insulin must be injected separately and not added to the mixture.

b. Alternately, the additional insulin can be given as type NPH, in 2 separate injections, spaced exactly 12 hours apart. N should not be mixed with UL, since N contains foreign proteins that are not present in UL. There may, therefore, be some allergic or other unexpected physiologic response to the injection of these new proteins into a patient who does not ordinarily take N; thus, the use of Lente insulin might be preferred.

3. If, as the illness proceeds, more L or N insulin is required, the 2 daily doses should be gradually increased, fol-

lowing the guidelines of step 2. If only UL is used, increases should be more gradual.

4. As the body's response to illness or infection subsides, low BG values will be encountered. These should be treated as indicated in Chapter 14. The sweets used in such treatment should be totaled each day. This total should then be multiplied by the BG calibration for the sweets used, to give the cumulative BG reduction for the day. This value is then divided by the BG calibration for 1 unit of insulin to get the number of units of insulin to be cut from the dose of intermediate- or long-acting insulin. The following example may clarify the procedure:

A patient recovering from an illness has been taking 2 additional daily doses of Lente insulin. He consumed a total of 10 sugar cubes in the past 24 hours and has thereby repeatedly returned BG to his target value. These cubes had each been calibrated at 13 mg/dl for this patient. One unit of R insulin will lower his BG by 30 mg/dl. Ten sugar cubes @ 13 mg/dl = 130 mg/dl, and 130 mg/dl ÷ 30 mg/dl per unit of insulin = 4 units insulin.

The patient now must reduce the extra Lente insulin by 4 units per day. He will, therefore, reduce each of his two supplementary doses of Lente by 2 units. Note that we are reducing his dose twice as rapidly as we raised it. That is, we did not cut the dosage reduction by ½, as we did with the dosage increase. This is to minimize the chances of hypoglycemia.

5. BG should still be monitored, with increased frequency, until total insulin dose has stabilized. There is always a possibility that the post-illness doses may stabilize above or below the pre-illness values.

6. Throughout the illness, additional doses of Regular insulin should be used to lower elevated BG as it occurs.

BG Control When Diet Has Been Reduced or Patient Is Not Eating

The important point to remember is that all insulin-dependent patients require insulin every day—even if not eating. The counter-regulatory processes are especially active when a patient is sick and fasting. In all likelihood, the basal or long-acting insulin doses will have to be supplemented, as indicated in the preceding section. The usual doses of Regular insulin will have to be reduced if the patient is eating less, or eliminated if the patient is not eating at all. Supplementary injections of Regular insulin must still be administered, whenever BG is elevated.

Even a reduced diet must still be planned and covered by Regular insulin. If meals are smaller and more frequent, doses of Regular insulin must also be smaller and more frequent. Simple sugars, including fruits, must still be excluded from the diet. Glucose or sucrose may, of course, be used for treating low BG.

How are preprandial doses of Regular insulin worked out when meal size is reduced? A good rule of thumb is to utilize a number that we call "effective grams of carbohydrate." *The effective grams of carbohydrate are simply the total of carbohydrate grams plus half the protein grams.* This number is computed for a reduced meal and divided by the effective grams of carbohydrate in a standard meal. The quotient is multiplied by the standard preprandial dose of Regular insulin, to get the reduced dose.

The following example demonstrates how this is done. Note that 1 ounce (28 grams) of lean meat contains only 7 grams of protein and therefore only $\frac{1}{2} \times 7 = 3\frac{1}{2}$ grams of effective CHO.

Reduced Meal		Effective grams CHO
2 oz. lean meat = 2 × 3.5 grams	=	7
⅓ bread exchange of vegetables = ⅓ × 12 grams	=	4
	Total	11

Standard Meal		Effective grams CHO
7 oz. lean meat = 7 × 3.5 grams	=	24.5
1 bread exchange of vegetables = 1 × 12 grams	=	12
	Total	36.5

Regular insulin for standard meal: 5 units
Regular insulin for reduced meal:

$$(11 \div 36.5) \times 5 \text{ units} = 1.5 = 1.5 \text{ units}$$

This formula is approximate and can be adjusted in the light of subsequent postprandial BG measurements.

Ketosis and Ketoacidosis

If the ill diabetic does not take enough insulin to offset the aforementioned counter-regulatory effects on BG, the BG may rise to the point where glucose can no longer enter insulin-dependent tissues and the energy metabolism of the body switches over to utilize fat as its principal source of fuel. The breakdown of fats in the liver leads to the production and accumulation in the blood of ketonic acids. These acids are detectable by their breakdown products, ketones, which can be measured in the urine. The presence of ketonic acids in the blood is called ketosis. If the acidity of the blood then increases beyond a certain point, we speak of keto-acidosis. As the body excretes glucose and toxic ketonic acids into the urine, the high urinary output (dehydration) draws along naturally occurring salts that would otherwise serve to neutralize additional ketonic acids. As a result, ketoacidosis is not self-limiting but gets worse as the patient becomes dehydrated. If the patient is already losing fluids through vomiting or diarrhea, as in many illnesses, ketoacidosis can proceed rapidly. Since the standard treatment of ketoacidosis includes the intravenous replacement of fluid and certain salts, hospitalization is usually required. A diabetic patient who has any illness that involves diarrhea, vomiting, or inability to eat should:

1. Contact his physician.
2. Test urine for ketones, every 3–4 hours.
3. Monitor BG at least every 2–3 hours.
4. Attempt to keep BG within target range agreed upon with physician.
5. Consume plenty of fluids, at a minimum rate to be specified by physician. Fluids can include sugar-free broth, boullion, soft drinks, very diluted tomato juice,[1] or tea. The physician may prescribe a certain number of *calibrated* sweets or sugar cubes to be dissolved in beverages and covered by small *calibrated* doses of Regular insulin, administered far enough in advance of drinking to prevent BG elevation. The added sweets can prevent starvation ketosis (described below) if BG remains normal. If vomiting or nausea makes it difficult to retain fluids, attempts should be made to feed only 1 tablespoon at a time, whenever the acute phase subsides. Fluids should not be forced. Alternately, it may be possible for the patient to get some fluid by sucking cracked ice. The physician may wish to terminate nausea/vomiting by prescribing prochlorperazine suppositories in small doses.
6. If living alone, arrange in advance for assistance in case of illness. A sick diabetic cannot safely lie in bed all day, without insulin, fluids, and BG measurement. If too weak to attend to these things, call someone who can come to help. If friends or neighbors are not available, keep handy the tele-

---

1. 1 cup of tomato juice contains over 10 grams CHO or nearly 1 bread exchange.

phone number of the local Visiting Nurse Service, Public Health Nursing Service, or Public Health Department. Their charges for such assistance are scaled according to income and are covered by Medicare, Medicaid, and health insurance plans.

If no foods are being consumed, *but BG remains normal*, there is still the possibility of developing starvation ketosis, as body fats are consumed for energy. This is a state that can also occur in fasting nondiabetics. It is not caused by high BG and should therefore not be confused with diabetic ketosis or ketoacidosis. Nevertheless, any positive test for urine ketones should be reported to the physician promptly. Starvation ketosis should not be allowed to continue for more than a few days, since ketones are toxic and their accumulation in blood and tissues can eventually be harmful. Furthermore, starvation ketosis can be accompanied by increased levels of counter-regulatory hormones (or reduced insulin binding) and can therefore cause BG elevation if not countered with additional insulin.

Oral Medications Containing Sugars

A cautionary note is necessary regarding medicines that contain sugar. Most cough medicines and many other forms of liquid oral medication, including liquid antibiotics, are basically unpleasant-tasting unless sweetened with some form of sugar, and should be avoided if possible. Alternate brands, that have been sweetened with saccharin, are frequently available and should be specified by physicians when writing prescriptions. Most pharmacists are familiar with any such alternates that may be available. An up-to-date list of sugar-free medicines sold in the U.S. is usually available at no charge, from The American Diabetes Association, 2 Park Avenue, New York, N.Y. 10016.

17

GETTING STARTED—A STEP-BY-STEP
SUMMARY

The reader, hopefully, has now digested the prior 16 chapters of this manual, as well as Appendix A and Appendix E, and the patient is ready to embark on the new regimen. To facilitate the planning of a program custom-tailored for each patient, we have provided the following checklist, which can serve as a guide simultaneously for both clinician and patient:

1. Secure necessary materials for the patient.
   a. A copy of this manual and the Joslin Diabetes Manual. A copy of *Food Values of Portions Commonly Used* is also highly recommended (see Appendix E).
   b. At least 100 DEXTROSTIX (page 69) and at least 25 CHEMSTRIP bG (page 71) reagent strips for measuring blood glucose.
   c. Hypodermic needles, or MONOLET lancets (page 77) with AUTOLET spring-driven lancet holder (page 77) for finger puncture.
   d. Appropriate insulin (usually U-100 Regular and Ultralente).
   e. Insulin syringes suitable for measuring small doses (usually ½-cc, disposable, U-100).
   f. Reflectance colorimeter for accurately reading reagent strips. We currently recommend any instrument (such as the Ames GLUCOMETER, etc.) that can be calibrated using at least two (high and low) liquid

glucose standards and checked for accuracy at normal BG, using a third liquid standard. But our preference may change as other instruments enter the market-place.

g. At least two sets (one for home, one for travel) of Ames DEXTRO-CHEK Calibrator (50 and 300 mg/dl glucose solutions). At least two vials of DEXTRO-CHEK 100 mg/dl control solution.

h. At least five copies of the GLUCOGRAF Data Sheet, and, if desired, of the Meal Composition Record. These can be photocopied from the removable insert (Figs. 16 and 17), located on pages 100–101 and 108–109, or can be purchased on pads (page 97).

i. An accurate scale for measuring body weight. To be used as a guide to appropriate size of protein and fat portions in meals and for fine-tuning dosage of Regular insulin (pages 160–161).

2. Perform optional baseline measurements for future comparisons (see Chapter 7). Typical tests might include:

a. Glycosylated hemoglobin (HbA_{1c} or HbA_1).

b. Urinary C-peptide in 24 hours (to assist in classifying the type of diabetes).

c. Renal function.
   (i) Quantitative urine protein (usually elevated when BG is chronically high, frequently returns to normal after an extended period of normal BG).
   (ii) Addis count.
   (iii) Creatinine clearance.
   (iv) B.U.N.

d. Lipid profile.
   (i) Serum cholesterol (total).
   (ii) Serum triglycerides.
   (iii) HDL cholesterol.

e. Nerve conduction velocities.

f. Quantitative fluorescein photometry of vitreous humor.

3. Patient learns technique for blood glucose measurement and proper use of Data Sheets. If using the discontinued EYETONE ® meter, consider the calibration method described in Appendix G.

4. Patient spends about 2 weeks perfecting BG monitoring technique and entering data onto Data Sheets. If patient has been testing urine, these tests should continue during this period only. He should also study basic diabetes texts (Appendix E), if necessary, as well as this manual. He should attempt to calibrate BG effects of sweets and of Regular insulin. This may not be possible, because BG may not yet be stable enough for calibrations to be valid.

5. After about 2 weeks, clinician reviews data sheets.

6. Clinician and patient agree on plans for maintenance or modification of body weight.

7. Clinician works out new schedule of insulin dosage (Chapter 12) and accompanying dietary recommendations. It is usually not wise to add a strenuous exercise program at this stage.

8. A date is set for starting the new regimen. It should coincide with a time when clinician is available for possible 24-hour-a-day telephone consultation for a period of at least 2 weeks.

9. Changeover to new regimen should be complete and instantaneous, covering all phases of diet and insulin dosage at once. Failure to execute a complete transition can be a major mistake. Clinician should exert special caution to ensure that dose of long-acting insulin is not excessive and approximates our guidelines. From this point on, postprandial hyperglycemia is to be controlled by Regular insulin plus diet.

10. Patient should be in daily telephone contact with clinician, for the purpose of discussing the minor changes in insulin and diet that are inevitable during the early period of adjustment (about 2 weeks). If, as suggested, Ultralente is

taken to wait at least 3 days between changes in dose of this insulin, unless it is causing frequent hypoglycemia.

11. After BG has stabilized within the target range, telephone contact can be reduced to cover only unusual situations, such as illness or travel. Calibration of Regular insulin and sweets should be complete.

12. Monthly visits to the clinician for routine blood and urine studies (glycosylated hemoglobin, etc.), review of Data Sheets, and planning of treatment are mandatory until the physician and patient are convinced that BG is being maintained essentially within the agreed target range.

13. In some cases, the initial target range for BG will, for the purpose of the patient's comfort, be higher than the 80–120 mg/dl suggested herein. Sooner or later the patient and clinician must agree to a timetable for changeover to the final target range. Once this range has been achieved, visits to physician's office or clinic may be cut back. Some physicians feel that if glycosylated hemoglobin can be maintained in the nondiabetic range, routine visits can be reduced to once every 3–6 months.

14. When clinician and patient are satisfied with stability and range of BG, it is appropriate to introduce a regular physical exercise program. For patients at high cardiac risk, the usual stress testing should precede the introduction of exercise. Plans should also be made for high-risk patients to ensure that physical exertion is built up according to a gradual predetermined schedule.

15. The first exercise period should include the calibration discussed in Chapter 15 and should be followed by a planned reduction in dosage of long-acting insulin.

16. Once BG has been stabilized within the target range, it is appropriate to calibrate the effects of Regular insulin when injected intramuscularly, observing the precautions cited on pages 137–138.

We hope that the detailed measures for normalizing BG that are described in this manual are not taken as absolute or unchangeable. There are probably many successful personally tailored variations that can be devised by creative health professionals or patients. The success of any variation can be estimated by answering the following questions:

a. Is HbA_{1c}[2] always within the nondiabetic range?

b. What fraction of patient-performed BG measurements (including those following meals) are within the target range?

c. Have episodes of hypoglycemia declined in frequency and severity and are physician, patient, and patient's family satisfied that any episodes of low blood sugar are so mild that there is no danger of loss of consciousness?

---

2. See footnote on page 61.

18

SOME PSYCHODYNAMIC
CONSIDERATIONS

Over the past thirty years, a "modern" philosophy of treatment for IDDM has evolved, that places major emphasis on preservation of a patient's "life style." It assumes that injecting insulin, testing urine, and restricting fancy desserts involve a great degree of personal sacrifice and serve to remind the patient continually that he has a chronic disease and is thus "different" from his peers. Advocates of this philosophy maintain that artificial regimentation of life style should be minimized, to enable the patient to feel that he is not different. Otherwise, he will have a negative self-image and will deteriorate emotionally. The concept of "not different" has repeatedly appeared in written material intended for the patient or his family and reminds one of a form of brainwashing. Another fictitious assumption encountered all too frequently is that multiple daily injections, frequent testing of urine or blood, and "exaggerated" interest in BG level will somehow turn the individual into a compulsive neurotic.

This philosophy ignores several basic points that are essential to the physical and emotional well-being of the insulin-dependent diabetic:

1. A person who feels chronically hungry, tired, thirsty, or weak knows, subconsciously, in spite of possible superficial denial, that he is sick. He will feel damaged and inadequate.

2. The diabetic woman who continually miscarries, or the impotent diabetic man (60 percent of all male diabetics are

at least partially affected), is not likely to have a positive self-image.

3. Most diabetics are fully aware of the statistics relating to long-term complications and many already suffer from some of the effects. Obviously this is going to cause depression, anxiety, and impaired body image. Ignoring the statistics serves no purpose, but preventing complications by proper treatment can certainly put many minds at rest.

4. The current data relating long-term complications to poor control of BG is quite clear (Chapter 2 and Appendix D). At the very least, the option of how much effort to be put into regulating BG should be up to the diabetic. If the decision to ignore these data is made by someone else, the problems cannot possibly be alleviated by the patient.

5. In the nondiabetic, BG is finely controlled over a narrow range, where the high end (perhaps 140 mg/dl) is about twice as great as the low end (perhaps 60 mg/dl). In IDDM, the high end (perhaps 600 mg/dl) is typically thirty times the value at the low end (perhaps 20 mg/dl). There is no doubt that diabetics can feel the effects of these BG extremes on their physiology. They know that such wide swings are "bad" but heretofore have usually been unable to control them. They are frustrated and imprisoned by the unpredictable whipsaw to which their metabolic state is continually subjected.

6. To tell an insulin-dependent diabetic that he is just like everyone else and can lead a normal life confuses him because it doesn't jibe with reality. He wishes that this were so and tends to believe the idealized authority figures (medical personnel) upon whom he is dependent. His bodily perceptions, however, tell him that he is not well and not normal. He thus may be disturbed by the conflict between the two sources of data and feels guilty for not feeling as healthy as he has been told he is. He may conclude, therefore, at some level, that the problem is in his mind and not in the real

world. Many bright and assertive diabetics say, "My doctor says I am fine, but why do I feel so terrible?" It is reassuring when these patients realize that, indeed, there is something wrong, that their diabetes controls many aspects of their lives, and that they must attend to their illness instead of ignoring it in order to feel well. It is better to be told what is wrong and to do all that is possible to set it right, than to be encouraged to ignore the true situation and its needs.

Group Training Sessions, Role Models, and Their Effects Upon Patients

There may be advantages to both physician and patients for people to be trained (in our regimen) in small groups, rather than individually. The problems that diabetics face are rarely understood by family members, and as a result many patients feel "alone" with their disease. Learning and comparing results with other patients can heighten enthusiasm and strengthen compliance. It also relieves the hopelessness that some patients experience when faced with what appears to be a monumental task.

The feasibility of convincing patients that they can do the job and will feel better, both physically and emotionally, can be enhanced by the occasional presence of a role model. The role model is simply a patient who is already practicing the regimen, and has begun to reap its benefits. Patients will often attach more credibility to the words of someone who has been in their position than to the promises of a professional.

The ideal size of training groups appears to be three to five patients. Larger groups may bring forth too many personal problems, and thereby slow down the training program.

The comments made by the diabetics in our group-training sessions bring to mind an experiment used in many elementary psychology courses. It illustrates the origins of much of the emotional effect that current, conventional approaches to treatment of IDDM have had on the patient:

A laboratory rodent is placed in a cage containing two buttons. One button releases a food pellet, the other creates a mildly painful electric shock. The animal rapidly learns to select the proper button when it is hungry, and manages eventually to get by without suffering electric shocks. After it has adjusted thoroughly to the experimenter's game, the rules are suddenly randomized. There is no longer any way for the animal to predict which button will excite which response. Of course, the animal rapidly becomes neurotic. Most insulin-dependent diabetics have, similarly, been taught an elaborate set of "logical" rules, relating to urine tests, effects of diet, use of insulin, etc. If these rules are followed, the patient is told, he will feel well and will be able to live a long, untroubled life. The patient is rarely advised that the rules, which have been in use so many years, just do not work. As a result, we see confusion, frustration, anger, self-blame, and similar responses to the unpredictable swings in blood sugar that buffet the patient. Feelings of despair, anxiety, guilt, helplessness, anger, resentment, and chronic depression often follow, as seen in the profiles in Chapter 4.

Patients who embark on our regimen are usually not extraordinarily motivated. They just want an opportunity to have control over their own metabolism. They feel that they are getting a good return for their dietary sacrifices and for their investment of perhaps 20 minutes daily in BG measurement and insulin administration. They also feel greater freedom by not being tied to the traditional rigid scheduling of meals and snacks.

Perhaps of greatest importance are the changes that eventually appear in the aspects of daily living that are supposedly unrelated to their diabetes. Relationships with family members usually improve. Job and educational careers frequently blossom and interactions with associates become less strained. It is as if, once an individual reaps the benefits of the order and harmony he has introduced into his diabetic state, he tends to bring order and harmony to other facets of life that have now taken on a new importance.

Appendix A

THE GLUCOGRAF LIST OF FOOD
EXCHANGES FOR DIABETICS

Prepared jointly with Judith Wylie-Rossett, Ed.D., R.D.
Director of Nutrition Training
The Diabetes Research and Training Center of
the Albert Einstein College of Medicine
and Montefiore Hospital & Medical Center

This appendix consists of three lists which cover a wide variety of food products for diabetic diets:

1. Milk products
2. Protein products
3. Vegetable products

We have tried to emphasize low-carbohydrate and low-fat products. Desserts and fruits have not been included because their high content of simple sugars rapidly raises blood glucose.

Bread and grain products, while common sources of B-complex vitamins, have not been included because they have high carbohydrate content. Furthermore, for the purpose of a sandwich, 1 standard 23-gram slice of white, rye, or whole-wheat bread has the carbohydrate content (12 grams) of 1 bread exchange (without the need of an exchange list). The following alternate sources of B-complex vitamins are recommended:

A variety of vegetables from the list of vegetable products beginning on page 233. Be sure to include green vegetables such as broccoli, spinach, or bean sprouts, which are very high in B-complex vitamins, or

One tablespoon daily of brewer's yeast, which contains about 4 grams of carbohydrate (one-third bread exchange), or

One B-complex vitamin capsule daily, containing from 50 percent to no more than 150 percent of the recommended daily allowances (RDA) for each of the B vitamins.

Readers interested in a far more complete listing of caloric, fat, CHO, protein, vitamin, mineral, and fiber values for several thousand foods should see *Food Values of Portions Commonly Used,* an important reference work listed in Appendix E.

PROTEIN PRODUCTS

Trim off visible fat. Pour off melted fats.

Two ounces (56 grams) of a low-fat protein product contain about 16 grams protein and have about the same (but much slower) effect upon blood glucose as 8 grams of carbohydrate or ⅔ bread exchange. See pages 160–168 for determination of protein portions.

Low-Fat Protein Products

Most people should select from this group in preference to the other two protein groups that follow.

BEEF

baby beef	flank	plate skirt steak	rump
chipped beef	tenderloin	round steak	tripe
chuck	plate ribs		

CHEESES

Any marked on label "contains less than 5 percent butterfat." Also see item number 7 on page 159.

EGGS

egg whites
EGG BEATERS (1 package also contains 1 bread exchange
of CHO) (Standard Brands, Inc., New York, N.Y. 10022).

FISH

fresh or frozen: all types, without added sauces or bread
crumbs

canned: mackerel, salmon, sardines (drained and blotted),
tuna (water-packed)

shellfish: (all types appear to contain substances—shellfish
sterols—that can lower serum cholesterol)

LAMB

leg	shank
loin (roast and chops)	shoulder
rib	sirloin

PORK

leg (center shank, whole rump)
ham
smoked center slices

POULTRY—skin removed

chicken	guinea hen	turkey
Cornish game hen	pheasant	

VEAL

cutlets	loin	shank
leg	rib	shoulder

Intermediate-Fat Protein Products

Most people should limit consumption to two or three times per week.

BEEF

corned beef, canned   rib eye
ground (15 percent fat)   round, ground, commercial

BEEF PARTS (high in cholesterol)

heart   liver
kidney   sweetbreads

CHEESE

farmer's   mozzarella   ricotta
Neufchatel   Parmesan

EGG

white, plus yolk (yolk is high in cholesterol)

PORK

Boston butt   ham, boiled   shoulder arm
Canadian bacon   loin (tenderloin) shoulder blade

High-Fat Protein Products

Most people should limit to special treats—perhaps once per week.

BEEF

brisket   ground (more than 20 per-
corned   cent fat)
                               hamburger, commercial
chuck, ground, commercial   rib steak
club steak   rib roasts

CHEESE, HARD	CHEESE, SEMI-SOFT	CHEESE, SOFT
cheddar type	bleu	Brie
Swiss type	brick type	Camembert
Gouda	munster	

LAMB

breast

PORK

ground	loin (back ribs)
ham, country style	sausage
ham, deviled	spare ribs

POULTRY

capon
duck
goose

SAUSAGE

bologna	salami
frankfurter	liverwurst

VEAL

breast

MILK PRODUCTS

Milk and cheese products are important sources of calcium. High-protein diets are usually high in phosphorus content. Since phosphorus intake should be balanced with calcium, it is wise to consume one serving of a milk or cheese product each day. This may be taken, for example, as ⅓ serving per meal. Children and pregnant or lactating women may require a higher intake of milk.

We have deliberately excluded from the following list milk products with high fat content.

1 fluid ounce = 2 tablespoonfuls   8 fluid ounces = 1 cup   1 ounce (avoirdupois) = 28 grams

	Serving Size	Carbohydrate		Protein (grams)	Fat (grams)
		Grams	Bread Exchange [2]		
Alba dairy light,[1] for coffee and tea	1 envelope	1	1/12	1	0
Buttermilk, fortified, skim, cultured	8 oz.	12	1	8	0–2
Cottage cheese, dry	4 oz. (½ 8-oz. pkg.)	2	1/6	16	0
Cottage cheese, half creamed, 2% butterfat	4 oz. (½ 8-oz. pkg.)	3	1/4	16	2
Milk, low fat, 1% fat	8 oz.	12	1	8	3
Milk, low fat, 1% fat with nonfat milk solids added	8 oz.	12	1	8	2
Milk, low fat, 1% fat, protein fortified	8 oz.	14	1	8	3
Milk, low fat, 2% fat	8 oz.	12	1	8	5
Milk, low fat, 2% fat, with nonfat milk solids added	8 oz.	12	1	8	5
Milk, low fat, 2% fat, protein fortified	8 oz.	14	1	8	5
Milk, nonfat (skim)	8 oz.	13	1	9	0
Milk, nonfat (skim), protein fortified	8 oz.	14	1	10	1
Yogurt, plain, made from low-fat milk	8 oz.	13	1	8	4

[1] Alba dairy light is the only currently acceptable packaged "creamer." All others contain sucrose or other simple sugars.

[2] The "bread exchange" is the basic unit of measure that we use for complex carbohydrate in our diet. It is based on the common 23-gram slice and *contains 12 grams of CHO.* This manual does not use the American Diabetes Association bread exchange, which is based upon a 27-gram slice and contains 15 grams of CHO. All carbohydrate-containing foods that appear in Appendix A are shown with their CHO content in grams and the equivalent bread exchange value.

VEGETABLE PRODUCTS

Vegetables are a very important component of the GLU-COGRAF diet. They contain vitamins and minerals and also add bulk or fiber to the diet. A high-protein diet containing a variety of vegetables and some milk products can be very nutritious.

This list is divided into six groups according to the amount of carbohydrate (CHO) in one serving as well as the approximate bread exchange:[1]

1	1/4
1/2	1/6
1/3	1/10

The low-carbohydrate vegetables are to be especially encouraged for several reasons. First, a greater variety can be eaten in the course of one day, providing a broader assortment of vitamins and minerals. Second, they provide greater bulk and therefore can be counted on to satisfy the appetite. Thus the judicious use of vegetables can aid in overcoming the habit of overeating, so common among insulin-dependent and overweight diabetics.

High-carbohydrate "starchy" vegetables, such as corn and potatoes, have been deliberately omitted from our lists. Potato does not appear for a second reason—when cooked it can raise BG almost as rapidly as pure glucose, because the high or prolonged cooking temperatures break its complex carbohydrates down to simple sugars.

---

1. The "bread exchange" is the basic unit of measure that we use for complex carbohydrate in our diet. It is based on the common 23-gram slice and *contains 12 grams of CHO*. This manual does not use the American Diabetes Association bread exchange, which is based upon a 27-gram slice and contains 15 grams of CHO. All carbohydrate-containing foods that appear in Appendix A are shown with their CHO content in grams and the equivalent bread exchange value.

Vegetable Product Servings

All serving sizes are ½ glass measuring cup (4 fluid ounces) unless otherwise indicated.

	Serving Size	Approximate Serving Weight (grams)
1. *About 10–13 grams CHO or 1 bread exchange per serving*		
Mixed vegetables, frozen, cooked, boiled, and drained		91
Peas, green, immature, raw, canned, or boiled and drained		72
Peas, green, and pearl onions, frozen, boiled and drained		94
Soybeans, cooked		90
2. *About 6–7 grams CHO or ½ bread exchange per serving*		
Artichoke bud, boiled, edible portion	½ large	60
Beets, red, boiled or canned, drained, sliced or diced		85
Carrot, raw, edible portion	1 medium	81
Rutabagas, cooked, boiled, drained, sliced or cubed		85
Tomatoes, cooked		120
3. *About 4–5 grams CHO or ⅓ bread exchange per serving*		
Asparagus, white, cut stalks, canned, drained		120
Beans, wax, cut, frozen, boiled and drained		67
Brussels sprouts, fresh or frozen		78
Carrots, cooked or canned, sliced or diced		75
Carrots, raw, grated or shredded		55
Collards, chopped frozen, boiled and drained		85
Eggplant, diced, boiled and drained		100
Kale, raw, leaves and stems, chopped		85
Kohlrabi, raw, diced		70
Mushrooms, fresh, or canned and drained		135
Okra pods, boiled and drained		80
Onion rings, frozen		14
Onions, French fried, canned		14
Sauerkraut, canned, solids and liquid		118
Tomato, ripe, raw or cooked	½ medium	75
Tomatoes, canned, solids and liquid		120
Turnips, cubed, raw or boiled and drained		72

	Serving Size	Approximate Serving Weight (grams)
4. *About 3–4 grams CHO or ¼ bread exchange per serving*		
Asparagus, green, fresh or frozen, whole stalks, boiled and drained		93
Asparagus, green, canned, cut stalks, drained		117
Bean sprouts (mung beans), boiled and drained		63
Beans, green, cut, canned or boiled and drained		66
Beans, green, frozen, cut, boiled and drained		63
Beans, green, raw, whole		55
Beans, wax, cut, canned or fresh, boiled and drained		65
Broccoli, fresh, chopped, boiled and drained		78
Cabbage, shredded, boiled and drained		72
Cauliflower, whole flowers, boiled and drained		63
Chard, Swiss, leaves, boiled and drained		88
Collards, leaves and stems, boiled and drained		72
Dandelion greens, boiled and drained, not packed in cup		52
Kale, leaves without stems and midribs, boiled and drained		55
Mustard greens, leaves without stems and midribs, boiled and drained		70
Onion, boiled and drained	½ medium	20
Spinach, fresh, frozen, or canned, boiled and drained		100
Squash, summer, sliced, boiled, and drained, all varieties		90
Tomato, raw	½ medium	75
Turnip greens, fresh or frozen, chopped, boiled and drained		77
5. *About 2 grams CHO or 1/6 bread exchange per serving*		
Beet greens, boiled and drained		72
Cabbage, raw, coarsely shredded or sliced		35
Cabbage, red, raw, coarsely shredded		35
Kale, leaves and stems, boiled and drained		55
Lettuce, Bibb or Boston, raw	½ head	82
Mustard greens, frozen, chopped, boiled and drained		75
Pepper, green sweet, empty shell, raw or cooked	¼ shell, or ¼ cup if chopped	82
Radishes, red, raw	5 small	50

	Serving Size	Approximate Serving Weight (grams)
6. About 2 grams CHO or 1/10 bread exchange per serving		
Artichoke hearts, deluxe, Bird's Eye	1 heart	16
Cabbage, boiled and drained	1 leaf	25
Cabbage, Chinese, raw, shredded	1 cup	44
Celery, raw, chopped or diced	¼ cup	30
Celery, raw, inner stalk	1 large	40
Chicory greens, raw	½ cup	13
Chives, raw, chopped	1 tablespoon	10
Cucumber, raw	½ medium	50
Endive, raw	5 long leaves, or 10 small leaves	25
Garlic, raw	1 clove	3
Lettuce, Bibb or Boston, raw	1 cup	55
Lettuce, iceberg, raw, shredded or chopped	1 cup	55
Lettuce, iceberg, raw, chunks	1 cup	75
Lettuce, iceberg, raw, leaves	1 cup	20
Lettuce, romaine, raw, shredded or chopped	1 cup	55
Lettuce, romaine, raw, leaf	½ cup	20
Mushrooms, fresh, raw (Agaricus)	5 small 2 large	50
Mushrooms, sautéed or fried (Lactarius)	4 medium	70
Onions, raw, chopped	1 tablespoon	10
Parsley, raw, chopped	1 tablespoon	10
Tofu (soybean curd), brick measures 2½″ × 2¾″ × 1″	½ brick	60
Watercress, raw	10 sprigs	10

Patients have been fairly creative in devising new recipes that add color and variety to our low CHO diet. The frequency of recipe exchanges at group training sessions has prompted us to plan a low CHO recipe book by diabetics and dietitians for diabetics. We are therefore soliciting contributions. Our initial guidelines encourage the use of low-fat protein products, high-fiber/low-carbohydrate vegetables, and polyunsaturated fats. The use of simple sugars, most fruits, starchy products, and high carbohydrate sweeteners such as fructose and sorbitol will be discouraged. Recipes may be mailed to:

Dr. Richard Bernstein
Diabetes Center
Albert Einstein College of Medicine
1300 Morris Park Avenue
Bronx, N.Y. 10461

A dietitian will review each recipe and will provide an analysis of protein, carbohydrate, saturated fat, and unsaturated fat breakdowns that will be published with each recipe. If possible, the recipes will also be tested. All submissions will be acknowledged but publication is not guaranteed. Authors will not be paid for their submissions but their names will be printed with their published recipes if specially requested in the letter of submission.

Appendix B

MANAGEMENT OF THE DIABETIC
UNDERGOING SURGERY

by Stephen B. Lewis, M.D.; Joel R. Poole, M.D.; James K. Schmitt, M.D.; Arie Maman, M.D.; and Michael M. Bliziotes, M.D.; Clinical Investigation Center, Naval Regional Medical Center, Oakland, California 94627

Note: The opinions or assertions contained herein are those of the authors and are not to be construed as official or as reflecting the views of the Navy Department or the naval service at large. This appendix is based on studies supported by funds provided by the Bureau of Medicine and Surgery, Navy Department, for CIP 5-48-387.

This appendix is included for the benefit of physicians who want to maintain their diabetic patients at or near normal blood glucose levels during and after surgery but have had no experience at such an undertaking. Although it is still common practice to keep BG elevated in diabetic surgical patients (to avoid hypoglycemia), the tide is beginning to turn. At the very least, patients who have taken the many steps toward BG control outlined in this manual will certainly expect a degree of care that approaches what they can achieve on their own, while they are totally in the hands of medical personnel.

Proper management of the diabetic patient about to undergo elective or emergency surgery is clouded in controversy. Disagreement among physicians concerning perioperative management centers on the methods used to obtain control of blood glucose, and the degree of control necessary. One group of physicians believes that strict control of blood glucose offers no demonstrable advantage. These feel that it is important only to avoid the extremes of hypoglycemia and hyperglycemia and the associated complications. We differ significantly from this view, in that our approach includes not only avoiding hypoglycemia and hyperglycemia, but also attempting to control blood glucose strictly within the range of 100–200 mg/dl during the perioperative period. Of course, the methods used to obtain this goal will vary, depending upon the type of anesthesia used, the clinical status of the patient during the perioperative period (for example, patient's weight), the presence of associated infection, renal insufficiency, or myocardial infarction, and the type of surgery.

We explain the rationale for our strategy of perioperative management and some of the ways by which we individualize therapy for each patient. Although most of the patients that we encounter have been on conventional 2 daily dose mixtures of Regular and NPH insulins,[1] we have in this appendix adapted procedures to patients who arrive well regulated on the 3-dose regimen described in Chapter 12.

Reasons for Strict Control

First, let us consider the potential risks involved should a surgical patient be allowed to remain hyperglycemic—here defined as serum glucose greater than 200 mg/dl. Unchecked hyperglycemia increases the potential for either ketoacidosis or hyperosmolar nonketotic coma.[2,3] We also know from animal studies and observation that other deleterious problems may arise as a result of persistent hyperglycemia:

1. Healing of surgical wounds is impaired.[4]
2. The patient's ability to combat infection may be ham-

---

1. Superior figures in this section refer to references at the end of this appendix.

pered both by diminished antibody response [5] and by impaired white blood cell action.[6]

3. Free fatty acids released into the circulation increase oxygen demand of the heart.[7,8]

4. An osmotic diuresis may cause fluid, electrolyte, and acid-base abnormalities.[9,10]

Strict control also means that we avoid hypoglycemia, which we here define as serum glucose less than 50 mg/dl. The risk of hypoglycemia during general anesthesia is increased since the signs and symptoms which accompany it are much less apparent. Frequent blood glucose monitoring by the anesthesiologist is therefore mandatory.

Many diabetics are apprehensive over the hazards of hypoglycemia or diabetic coma during surgery. This is especially true if a patient has been in full control of his own blood glucose levels and must turn over that control to someone of unknown competence. Much anxiety can be prevented if the patient is assured of a routine procedure for maintaining blood glucose within reasonable limits.

Approaches to Surgery

Having given our rationale for strict control, we wish to review, in a general way, our approach to a diabetic patient about to undergo surgery. Keep in mind that each patient's care must be individualized.

Outpatient Surgery

First, we will consider an example of an insulin-dependent diabetic who is to have outpatient dental surgery. For the purpose of discussion we will assume good control up to the day preceding surgery. We ask that the diabetic patient be given priority as the first case of the morning to avoid unnecessarily prolonged fasting. We recommend the following guidelines for this situation.

1. On the day prior to surgery, the patient receives the usual insulin dosages and eats the usual diet.

2. The patient fasts after midnight.

3. The diabetic is instructed not to take the usual pre-breakfast dose of short-acting (Regular) insulin. The usual doses of long-acting (for example, Ultralente) or intermediate-acting (for example, NPH) insulins should be administered.

4. On the morning of surgery, the patient measures blood glucose (BG).

    a. If BG exceeds 130 mg/dl, patient administers Regular insulin in accord with his usual calibration so that BG will be brought down to the middle of his target range, or to 100 mg/dl, whichever is higher.

    b. If BG is below 100 mg/dl, patient must eat calibrated glucose or sucrose tablets or powder to bring BG back up to at least 100 mg/dl. No complex carbohydrate, fruits, or fruit juices may be used for this purpose. Furthermore, at least 2 hours must elapse after such an event before anesthesia is administered.

    c. Should the blood glucose be greater than 300 mg/dl, surgery is cancelled until such time as good control is regained.

5. Following surgery which has otherwise proceeded uneventfully, blood glucose is monitored every 3 hours. Regular insulin or sweets (dissolved in liquid if a dental patient) are administered by the patient if necessary for maintaining BG within the target range.

Postoperatively, for the first day or two, the patient is provided with easily digestible meals, consisting principally of complex carbohydrate (CHO) and each covered by a dose of Regular insulin based upon the patient's usual calibrations for effects of bread exchanges (12-gram) on BG. We like to see adult patients consume up to 200 grams of CHO (800 calories) during each of these days. This can be divided between 4–8 small meals, depending upon the patient's tolerance for CHO. Type Ia diabetics (no endogenous insulin) may require 8 small snacks, each containing 18 grams, for a total of only 144 grams CHO for the day. If for any reason the patient is unable to tolerate this regimen, he or she is hospitalized for intravenous infusion of 5 percent dextrose in Ringer's Lactate (physiological salt solution)—to prevent starvation ketosis—and blood glucose monitoring. During the first two days, subcutaneous doses of long- or intermediate-acting insulins are maintained at preoperative levels.

Inpatient Surgery

Those patients requiring hospitalization are cared for by a team consisting of an internist/diabetologist, anesthesiologist, and surgeon—all working with the goal of maintaining serum glucose between 100–200 mg/dl during the perioperative period. The management during the day preceding surgery is similar to that of the outpatient who undergoes surgery.

We use either a Yellow Springs INSTRUMENT GLUCOSE ANALYZER—model 23A, range 0–500 mg/dl ± 2 mg/dl, requiring a 25 microliter blood sample—or an Ames DEXTROMETER reflectance meter, to monitor blood glucose. Either instrument properly calibrated can be used by patient, nursing personnel, or physician. The Ames instrument may be used in the presence of explosive anesthetics, provided it is powered by a battery pack and not by an alternating current line cord. The Yellow Springs instrument should not be used near explosive gases.

We recommend the following regimen for inpatient diabetic surgical cases:

1. On the day prior to surgery the patient receives the usual insulin dosage and eats the usual diet.

2. The patient fasts after midnight.

3. The diabetic is instructed not to take the usual pre-breakfast dose of Regular insulin, but the regimen of long- or intermediate-acting insulin is retained.

4. Upon induction of anesthesia, a constant intravenous dextrose infusion (via a Harvard pump) begins at a rate of 100 mg/kg/hour in order to reduce fat and protein breakdown. The dextrose is infused as a 5 percent solution in Ringer's lactate.

5. The anesthesiologist measures blood glucose at 15–30 minute intervals throughout the period of anesthesia.

6. Plain Ringer's Lactate is administered intravenously (via a second Harvard pump) at 4–10 mg/kg/hour, depending on the patient's fluid requirements during surgery.

7. Constant Regular insulin infusion by a third Harvard pump according to the algorithm of the following Table I. Insulin is fed to the pump from a plastic bag containing 250 ml of 155mM sodium chloride to which are added 50 units of U-100 regular pork insulin. (Pork insulin is used because about 10 percent of patients now use pork insulin, and introduction of mixed pork/beef insulin to these individuals could precipitate an immune response to insulin that can upset BG regulation for a number of months.) To saturate insulin binding sites within the plastic tubing, the first 75 ml of saline-insulin solution is flushed and discarded before connection to the indwelling intravenous line.

8. Should hypoglycemia occur, 12 ml of 50 percent dextrose (6 grams) is administered by bolus for a (60 ± 10 kg) patient.

9. For exceptional cases that fail to respond to the 20 units/hour Regular insulin infusion, we use the alogorithm of Table II.

Table I. Insulin Infusion Algorithm

Serum Glucose mg/dl	Regular Insulin units/hour	Glucose (5 percent dextrose) mg/kg/hour
Less than 100	0	100
100 to 200	1	100
Greater than 200	20	100

Table II. Insulin Bolus Algorithm

Serum Glucose mg/dl	Regular Insulin units/kg body weight
200–249	0.1
250–299	0.2
300–349	0.3
Greater than 350	0.4

To demonstrate the fact that patient's care must be individualized, we recently admitted to the hospital a (120-kg) patient, previously treated on a conventional insulin/diet regimen, who was septic from a gangrenous leg and in heart failure. These factors necessitated intravenous Regular insulin infusion at 40 units/hour. In addition, two additional intravenous boluses of 24 units Regular insulin were required at ½-hour intervals according to Table II. To maintain strict glucose control, 1 unit/hour Regular insulin infusion was required for an additional day postoperatively. In other instances, we have treated patients effectively with ½ unit/ hour.

Postoperative Care

Postoperatively, we continue with glucose/Regular insulin infusion or bolus (Table I or II), with blood glucose measurements every 1–3 hours, depending on the stability of the patient's diabetes. The intravenous route is selected because it provides the most direct route for delivery of insulin and glucose. In a 70-kg patient, this approximates 150 grams of glucose (or 3 liters of any 5 percent dextrose solution) and 24 units of Regular insulin in 24 hours. At no point is the patient's prior twice (in some cases thrice) daily regimen of subcutaneous injection of long- or intermediate-acting insulin interrupted.

When the patient is able to resume oral intake, we would shift to the insulin and complex CHO feeding regimen described at the end of the previous section on outpatient surgery. BG monitoring at least every 3 hours continues, with correction of high or low blood sugars according to the patient's presurgical routine.

The physician is immediately alerted if there is any sudden increase in insulin requirements. If this occurs, one begins an immediate search for infection, phlebitis, or silent myocardial infarction.

Postoperative glucose monitoring continues as usual after the patient is released. If problems occur, the patient is instructed to contact a team physician by phone. Routinely, the patient is scheduled for a follow-up visit to see his or her physician within a week after hospital discharge.

Summary

We believe that strict control of blood glucose is as important during the perioperative period as it is during routine outpatient management. Advantages of this approach include better surgical wound healing, higher resistance to infection, improved physiological adaptation of the patient's body to surgical stress, and reduction of anxiety.

References

1. Woodruff, R.E.; Lewis, S.B.; McLeskey, C.H.; and Graney, W.F. Avoidance of Surgical Hyperglycemia in Diabetic Patients, *JAMA* 244:166–168 (1980).

2. Feig, P.U., and McCurdy, D.K. The Hypertonic State, *N Engl J Med.* 289:843 (1973).

3. Foker, P. Hyperosmolar Hyperglycemic Nonketotic Coma: A Cause of Delayed Recovery from Anesthesia, *Anesthesiology* 41:284 (1974).

4. Goodson, W.H., III, and Hunt, T.K. Studies of Wound Healing in Experimental Diabetes Mellitus, *J Surg Res.* 22:221 (1977).

5. Bates, G., and Weiss, C. Delayed Development of Antibody to Staphylococcus Toxin in Diabetic Children, *Am J Dis Child.* 62:346 (1941).

6. Nolan, C.M.; Beaty, H.N.; and Bagdade, J.D. Further Characterization of the Impaired Bactericidal Function of Granulocytes in Patients with Poorly Controlled Diabetes, *Diabetes* 27:889 (1978).

7. Wahlqvist, M.L.; Kaijser, L.; Lassers, B.W.; *et al.* Fatty Acid as a Determinant of Myocardial Substrate and Oxygen Metabolism in a Man at Rest and during Prolonged Exercise, *Acta Med Scan.* 193:89 (1973).

8. Kjekshus, J.K.; Mjos, O.D. Effect of Free Fatty Acids on Myocardial Function and Metabolism in Ischemic Dog Heart, *J Clin Invest.* 51:1767 (1972).

9. Knochel, J.P. The Pathophysiology and Clinical Characteristics of Severe Hypophosphatemia, *Arch Interm Med.* 137:203 (1977).

10. Alberti, K.G.M.M.; Emerson, P.M.; Darley, J.H.; *et al.* 3-Diphosphoglycerate and Tissue Oxygenation in Uncontrolled Diabetes Mellitus, II, *Lancet* 2:391 (1972).

11. Lewis, S.B.; Wallin, J.D.; Kuzuya, H.; *et al.* Circadian Variation of Serum Glucose, C-Peptide Immunoreactivity, and Free Insulin in Normal and Insulin-Treated Diabetic Pregnant Subjects, *Diabetologia* 12:343 (1976).

Appendix C

HOME BLOOD-GLUCOSE MONITORING
(EDITORIAL)

by Dr. R. B. Tattersall

General Hospital, Nottingham, England

Reprinted by permission from
Diabetologia 16:71–74 (1979)
the journal of the European Association for the Study of
Diabetes

Diabetologia 16, 71–74 (1979)

Diabetologia

© by Springer-Verlag 1979

A recent review in this journal summarized the impressive evidence that poor control is one of the major factors responsible for the micro-vascular complications of diabetes [1]. If we accept this proposition, then it follows that diabetologists and their patients must make "a serious effort to achieve blood-glucose levels as close to those in the non-diabetic state as possible" [2], so long as this does not involve an unacceptably high risk of hypoglycaemia or a life style which will damage the patient psychologically.

Until the advent of automatic implantable devices, the only way of controlling insulin-dependent diabetes is for the patient to do it himself. Diabetics, unlike patients in most other areas of medicine, have always been given much responsibility for their own treatment and have been expected to carry out tasks such as injections and urine testing which are traditionally the preserve of professionals. In order to control his diabetes successfully the patient needs not only to be educated and motivated, but also to have a reliable means of monitoring his progress so that he can decide when and how to adjust insulin and diet.

Table 1. Publications on home blood glucose monitoring

Authors	System	Number of patients	Age range (years)
Sönksen et al. [8]	Eyetone	64	15–53
Walford et al. [9]	Reflomat	69	14–65
Danowski and Sunder [10]	Eyetone	5	11–24
Peterson et al. [11]	Eyetone	10	Mean 25
Ikeda et al. [12]	Eyetone	8	18–46
Skyler et al. [13]	Eyetone	32	Not specified

As a means of self monitoring, urine tests have always been unsatisfactory. They often do not reflect prevailing blood-glucose concentrations accurately [3] but their most serious drawback is that they give no information on blood-glucose fluctuations below the level of the renal threshold. This leads patients to equate negative urine tests with impending hypoglycaemia. The problem of the renal threshold also means that urine tests cannot be used to monitor strict control.

Renewed interest in strict diabetic control, the inadequacy of urine testing, and the traditional concept of giving the diabetic patient the responsibility for his own management, have led logically to the development of blood sugar measurement by patients themselves. The idea is not new. As long ago as 1962 Keen and Knight [4]

---

1. Figures in brackets refer to references at the end of this appendix.

showed that their patients could take a sample of capillary blood onto a filter paper which was then delivered to the hospital for analysis. Although this made it possible to measure blood sugars outside hospital, and incidentally showed how poorly controlled most patients were [5], it was unsatisfactory because it did not give instant results. Similar techniques which do not require the patient to be lent expensive equipment have recently been re-investigated and found to be accurate enough for clinical purposes [6, 7]. However, any method which does not give an immediate answer is unsatisfactory for the insulin-taking patient who needs to be able to act on the results.

Home blood-glucose monitoring has been made possible by the development of glucose oxidase based reagent strips and reflectance meters[1]. Six groups have now reported their experience in teaching insulin-treated diabetics to measure their own blood-glucose concentrations with a reflectance meter [8–13] (Table 1). Although these trials have differed in detail, the general conclusions have been remarkably similar. In summary these are:

1. That patients have little difficulty in pricking their fingers.

2. That the results which patients obtain are sufficiently accurate for ordinary clinical practice.

3. That self-monitoring of blood-glucose levels leads to increased motivation and better control in the majority of patients.

Obtaining the Blood Sample

Diabetic patients are used to needles and find little difficulty in pricking their fingers. Semi-automatic devices are available [14] but are rarely necessary. Although home blood-glucose monitoring has been used for paediatric patients [13] it is probably unreasonable to expect children

below the age of 12 to obtain the blood sample themselves. Either blood lancets or disposable needles can be used; patients find either "Monolets" or ⅜ × 26 gauge disposable needles most satisfactory. Teaching a patient to use a reflectance meter takes about 30 minutes and it is useful for either the doctor or nurse to demonstrate the technique on themselves, since this not only ensures that the machine is working and correctly standardized but also has a considerable psychological impact on the patient.

Accuracy

Both the Dextrostix-Eyetone and Reflotest-Reflomat systems give accurate results in the hands of experienced personnel [15, 16], although there is some divergence from autoanalyser results when the blood-glucose exceeds 12 mmol/l (216 mg/100 ml). Two groups [9, 12] have also found a close correlation between blood-glucose values obtained by patients themselves and simultaneous laboratory determinations. However, although this shows that patients *can* use the machine accurately, it does not prove that they will do so in practice. The best guarantee of accuracy lies in careful instruction of patients by someone who is fully conversant with the technique. Although it is probably easier to teach intelligent patients to use a meter, both Sönksen [8] and Walford [9] and their co-workers found that compliance and accuracy were by no means confined to higher socioeconomic classes or more intelligent patients.

Improved Motivation and Control

Direct measurement of blood-glucose levels has the great advantage over urine testing that the information "makes sense" to patients who may previously have performed urine tests conscientiously but without really understanding what they meant. Eighty percent of patients in one series thought that measuring their blood

---

1. Dextrostix-Eyetone system (Ames Corporation). Reflotest Reflomat system (Boehringer, Mannheim)

glucose was "a great help" and none found it of no benefit [8]. A high proportion of patients who have experienced home blood-glucose monitoring would prefer to continue with it rather than returning to urinanalysis [8, 13].

Control has been considerably improved in most patients who have monitored their own blood-glucose levels although some of this improvement may be due to the increased interest of both doctors and patients. It is also probable that some of the improvement results from better dietary compliance since many patients who monitor their own blood-glucose levels show improved control without changing their insulin dose [13]. In the study of Sönksen et al. [8] the mean clinic blood glucose fell from 11.8 to 8.9 mmol/l and two thirds of the patients were able to maintain a level of control in which 80% of their blood glucose values were below 10 mmol/l for periods exceeding a year. At the end of the Nottingham study [9] half the patients had glucose profiles in which no more than one of ten blood glucose determinations in a single day exceeded 10 mmol/l. The results achieved by Danowski and Sunder [10] and Peterson et al. [11], albeit on smaller and more selected groups, are even more impressive. In the former study five patients, aged 11 to 25 years, measured their blood-glucose levels 23 times a week and were able to maintain almost all values between 3 and 8 mmol/l for over a year. In the latter study 10 patients made measurements at least six times every day and adjusted their insulin accordingly. The mean Hb_{Alc} at the beginning of the study was 10.3% whereas after four to six months this had fallen to 5.4%.

It has been suggested [17] that strict control is likely to be accompanied by an increased frequency of hypoglycaemic reactions. This has not been the experience in trials of self monitoring of blood glucose. In the St. Thomas's series [8], 34% of patients had fewer, 46% the same frequency and 20% more hypoglycaemic reactions. It seems probable that severe hypoglycaemic reactions, often without warning symptoms, occur most often in patients who have excessive blood-glucose fluctuations rather than in patients who are strictly controlled. Self-monitoring is a particularly useful means of solving problems in patients who are having hypoglycaemic reactions [9], and is also useful in confirming the presence of a low blood-glucose level in patients whose symptoms might be due either to anxiety or hypoglycaemia [13]. Confirmation of hypoglycaemia is easy with a standard Dextrostix although with the Boehringer system it is necessary to use a separate stick (Reflotest hypoglycaemie) which has a range from 0.5 to 8 mmol/l.

Frequency of Testing

How often patients measure their blood sugars depends on the reason for which monitoring is undertaken. In the Nottingham study [9] which was devised primarily to obtain information about and improve the control of brittle diabetics, measurements were made approximately every hour and profiles obtained on two successive days, usually one working and one rest day. Others [8, 13] have used measurements four times daily: before each of the main meals and before going to bed. Preprandial or fasting measurements considerably underestimate the size of postprandial blood glucose peaks and are probably insufficient for monitoring the pregnant diabetic or attempting to achieve "super" control in the juvenile diabetic. In these cases the best results seem to be obtained by frequent determinations of blood glucose with multiple injections of insulin. A good compromise for long-term monitoring is the protocol advocated by Danowski and Sunder [10] in which patients measured a fasting and one other blood glucose on six out of the seven week days with a full profile on the 7th day which included determinations in the fasting state, before and after each meal and one blood glucose during the night.

R. B. Tattersall: Home Blood Glucose Monitoring

Advantages and Disadvantages of Self-Monitoring of Blood Glucose

The advantages of home blood-glucose monitoring are:

1. That it gives information about the pattern of blood-glucose fluctuations while patients are going about their ordinary life.

2. It enables the physician to advise on changes of treatment, over the telephone if necessary, on the basis of solid information. It eliminates the need to admit patients to hospital for stabilisation.

3. Patients are motivated and become more active partners in their own management.

Home blood-glucose monitoring is complementary to rather than a substitute for measurement of Hb_{Alc}. The latter, unlike home blood-glucose monitoring, does not depend on the patient's cooperation or accuracy. Furthermore, it provides a way of assessing diabetic control as a single number and is a useful end point at which to direct treatment [18]. The disadvantage is that it does not indicate *how* treatment should be changed to obtain better control. Thus, in many ways home blood-glucose monitoring and Hb_{Alc} measurement each supplement the defects of the other and should be regarded as complementary investigations. A study using both techniques on the same patients should make it possible to decide how much deviation from normoglycaemia is compatible with a normal Hb_{Alc} value.

A potential problem with home blood-glucose monitoring is that it might have adverse psychological effects by causing patients to be preoccupied with measuring their blood-glucose levels to the exclusion of a normal life. I have encountered this problem with one patient although it is only fair to say that he had previously been an obsessional urine tester! Generally home blood-glucose monitoring seems to improve a patient's psychological state rather than the converse. Patients who have difficulty in controlling their diabetes often develop a negative self-concept and a sense of hopelessness [19]. Home blood-glucose monitoring usually leads to in-

creased self-confidence and emotional stability which patients attribute to relief at being in control of their own physiology and no longer at the mercy of seemingly random processes [11].

The Future

The present capital cost of machines and sticks is such that most hospitals will have to use them selectively and sparingly. Home blood-glucose monitoring is clearly superior to other methods of assessing day-to-day control and should be regarded as a sine qua non for the management of diabetic pregnancy. For most other diabetic patients a meter is only necessary intermittently to check control or solve particular problems [9, 13]. If cheaper and more portable machines become available in the future, patients with brittle diabetes, and perhaps even every newly diagnosed insulin-taking diabetic, will benefit from doing regular blood test rather than urine tests.

The presently available Reflectance Meters were not designed for patient use and are bulky, mains operated, insufficiently robust and too expensive. The second generation of machines which have recently been marketed are not only cheaper but also more convenient. Both[2] are portable and have rechargeable batteries, a digital display, and built-in timer. If the initial impression that patients prefer blood to urine tests [8, 13] is substantiated, increased production will lead to still smaller and cheaper machines.

Conclusion

Doctors find it impossible to stabilize and monitor diabetic patients in hospital without measuring blood-glucose levels and it seemed logical that patients would also manage themselves better if they were

---

2 Glucocheck (Medistron Ltd., Crawley, Sussex, England and Hypo-Count (Hypoguard, Ipswich, England)

able to measure blood glucose during their ordinary life. The development of glucose oxidase sticks and Reflectance meters has made this possible. Six groups have published their experience with home blood-glucose monitoring in 188 patients. All have found their patients have little difficulty in obtaining blood samples and can get accurate results. When patients measure blood rather than urinary glucose they understand the disease better and become more motivated. Control has been greatly improved in the majority of patients and some can maintain normoglycaemia for long periods of time. Cheaper and more portable machines will make the method more widely applicable. Both Hb_{Alc} and home blood-glucose monitoring will be increasingly used in the management of the insulin-taking diabetic since they provide complementary information.

References

1. Tchobroutsky, G.: Relation of diabetic control to development of microvascular complications. Diabetologia 15, 143–152 (1978)
2. Cahill, G. F., Etzwiler, D. D., Freinkel, N.: 'Control' and diabetes. N. Engl. J. Med. 294, 1004–1005 (1977)
3. Malone, J. I., Rosenbloom, A. L., Grgic, A., Weber, F. T.: The role of urine sugar in diabetic management. Am. J. Dis. Child. 130, 1324–1327 (1976)
4. Keen, H., Knight, R. K.: Self sampling for blood sugar: Lancet 1962 I, 1037–1040
5. Beidas, A. S., Macfie, J. M., Morton, E. B. V., Wells, M. V.: Measurement of the blood glucose profile in diabetics by a self sampling technique. Paper presented at the 5th Congress of the International Diabetes Federation 1964
6. Wakelin, K., Goldie, D. J., Hartog, M., Robinson, A.P.: Measurement of capillary blood glucose in filter paper spots: An aid to the assessment of diabetic control. Br. Med. J. 1978 II, 468 –469
7. Howe-Davis, S., Holman, R. R., Phillips, M., Turner, R. C.: Home blood sampling for plasma glucose assay in control of diabetes. Br. Med. J. 1978 II, 596–598
8. Sönksen, P. H., Judd, S. L., Lowy, C.: Home monitoring of blood glucose. Lancet 1978 I, 729–732
9. Walford, S., Gale, E. A. M., Allison, S. P., Tattersall, R. B.: Self monitoring of blood glucose. Lancet 1978 I, 732–735
10. Danowski, T. S., Sunder, J. H.: Jet injection of insulin during self monitoring of blood glucose. Diabetes Care 1, 27–33 (1978)
11. Peterson, C. M., Jones, R. L., Dupuis, A., Bernstein, R., O'Shea, M.: Feasibility of tight control of juvenile diabetes through patient-monitored glucose determinations. Diabetes 27 [Suppl. 2], 437 (1978)
12. Ikeda, Y., Tajima, N., Nimami, N., Ide, Y., Yoroyama, J., Abe, M.: Pilot study of self-measurement of blood glucose using the Dextrostix-Eyetone System for juvenile onset diabetes. Diabetologia 15, 91–93 (1978)
13. Skyler, J. S., Lasky, I. A., Skyler, D. L., Robertson, E. G., Mintz, D. H.: Home blood glucose monitoring as an aid in diabetes management. Diabetes Care 1, 150–157 (1978)
14. Turner, R. C., Holman, R. R.: Automatic lancet for capillary blood sampling, Lancet 1978 II, 712
15. Jarrett, R. J., Keen, H., Hardwick, C.: "Instant" blood sugar measurement using Dextrostix and a reflectance meter. Diabetes 19, 724–726 (1970)
16. Brunton, W. A. T., Steele, J. M., Percy-Robb, I. W.: An assessment of a reflectance meter system for measurement of plasma or blood glucose in the clinic or side ward. Clin. Chim. Acta 75, 359–364 (1977)
17. Siperstein, M. D., Foster, D. W., Knowles, H. C., Levine, R., Maddison, L. L., Roth, J.: Control of blood glucose in diabetic vascular disease. N. Engl. J. Med. 296, 1060–1062 (1977)

18. Gonen, B., Rubenstein, A. H.: Hae-
    moglobin A1 and diabetes mellitus.
    Diabetologia **15**, 1–8 (1978)

19. Bruhn, J. G.: Self-concept and the
    control of diabetes. Am. Fam. Physi-
    cian **15**, 93–97 (1977)

Dr. R. B. Tattersall
Consultant Physician
Nottingham General Hospital
Nottingham NG1 6HA
England

Appendix D

BLOOD GLUCOSE CONTROL IN DIABETES

Reprinted from *Diabetes*
the journal of the American Diabetes Association, Inc.
Copyright 1976 by the American Diabetes Association, Inc.
25: no. 3:237–39 (March 1976)

ORGANIZATION SECTION

This policy statement of the American Diabetes Association is intended to publicize the belief that the weight of evidence, particularly that accumulated in the past five years,[1] strongly supports the concept that the microvascular complications of diabetes are decreased by reduction of blood glucose concentrations.

For almost 50 years, since insulin therapy was initiated, proponents of "rigid," "tight," or "chemical" control quoted retrospective evidence of decreased or delayed nephropathy and retinopathy as glucose levels are brought by therapy toward the normal range. Opponents to this hypothesis pointed to the problems of complications in many of these supposedly better-controlled patients, to the emotional and socioeconomic conflicts which often resulted from the demands of rigorous control, to the frequent difficulties with hypoglycemic reactions, and, recently, to the University Group Diabetes Project.[2,3]

Five years ago, in a review of 300 reports in the world literature evaluating control, Knowles[4,5] found data from 85 centers which were satisfactory for analysis. There were no prospective studies which proved or disproved that control prevented complications, and definite studies had yet to be done. He concluded that better means must be developed to achieve control than those presently available.

The University Group Diabetes Project was initiated to help settle the controversy. The five forms of therapy failed to demonstrate any effect upon microvascular lesions.[2,3] The middle-aged or older subjects studied exhibited only minimal initial hyperglycemia, however, and the reduction in blood glucose was small, so the results are not directly pertinent to the relationships between glucose levels and microvascular lesions.

In the past few years, numerous studies in animals, including dogs, rats, monkeys, Chinese hamsters, mice, and others, have demonstrated that reduction of hyperglycemia by insulin therapy, by transplantation of insulin-producing tissues, or by other means, prevents or minimizes formation of diabetic-like lesions in eye, kidney, and nerve.[1] Biochemical studies have shown persistent hyperglycemia to be associated with accumulation of sorbitol in nerve, eye, and vascular tissue and with alterations in vascular basement membrane.[6] Most recently, even hemoglobin has been found altered in man and experimental animals in the presence of persistent and prolonged hyperglycemia.[7-11]

Biopsies of kidney (and in some studies of muscle) have failed to show abnormalities for the first few years of insulin-dependent diabetes in man,[12-14] excluding thereby an independently inherited phenomenon. In a small but prospective study

---

1. Superior numbers refer to references at end of this appendix.

of randomly assigned patients just reported from Paris,[15] enthusiastically well-controlled diabetic subjects showed less retinopathy. Thus, the contention that the microvascular complications occur independently of the hyperglycemia and insulin deficiency and that control of the metabolic events is not a factor in their progress does not appear tenable any longer.

These data therefore place the burden of proof upon those who maintain that diabetes control is without effect. The goals of appropriate therapy should thus include a serious effort to achieve levels of blood glucose as close to those in the nondiabetic as feasible. Obviously, patient needs and resources must also be carefully assessed and the goals individualized accordingly. This concept is particularly applicable to the diabetics at greatest risk of developing the microvascular complications—the young and the middle-aged. It is well appreciated, however, that in some juvenile-onset-type subjects, it is most difficult, even with multiple insulin injections, to achieve any significant degree of control of the hyperglycemia. Also, in certain elderly patients, the shorter life expectancy may preclude the need for achieving lower glucose levels, providing they are asymptomatic.

In summary, current clinical and experimental data clearly demonstrates that optimal regulation of glucose levels should be achieved in the treatment of diabetes particularly in young and middle-aged individuals who are at greatest risk of developing the microvascular complications.

It can be concluded that current means of therapy are only partly effective at best, and therefore a high priority must be assigned to the development of more physiologic insulin delivery systems or to approaches to the correction of the deficient insulin-producing mechanism itself. Finally, good diabetic management necessitates education and training of both patients and health professionals in the technics involved, and close coordination and cooperation in patient management. Most important is a commitment to the view that better "control," when achievable, is beneficial.

REFERENCES

[1]Crofford, O., et al.: Reports to Congress of the National Commission on Diabetes. U. S. Government Printing Office, Public Law 93-354, 93rd Congress, S-2830, July 23, 1974. Findings and Declaration of Purpose Sec. 2(a)(3), 1975.

[2]University Group Diabetes Program. Effects of hypoglycemic agents on vascular complications in patients with adult-onset diabetes. III. Clinical implications of USDP results. J.A.M.A. 218:1400–10, 1971.

[3]University Group Diabetes Program. A study of the effects of hypoglycemic agents on vascular complications in patients with adult-onset diabetes. V. Evaluation of phenformin therapy. Diabetes 24 (Suppl. 1): 65–184, 1975.

[4]Knowles, H. C., Jr.: Control of Diabetes and the Progression of Vascular Disease in Diabetes Mellitus: Theory and Practice. Ellenberg, M. and Rifkin, H., Eds. New York, McGraw-Hill, 1970, Chapter 28, pp. 666–73.

[5]Knowles, H. C., Jr.: Long-term juvenile diabetes treated with unmeasured diet. Trans. Assoc. Am. Phys. 84–95, 1971.

[6]Spiro, R. G.: Biochemistry of renal glomerular basement membrane and its alterations in diabetes mellitus. N. Engl. J. Med. 228:1337–42, 1973.

[7]Trivelli, L. A., Ranney, H. M., and Lai, H. T.: Hemoglobin components in patients with diabetes mellitus. N. Engl. J. Med. 284:353–57, 1971.

[8]Bunn, H. F., Haney, D. N., Kamin, S., Gabbay, K., and Gallop, P.: The biosynthesis of human hemoglobin A_{Ic}: slow glycosylation of hemoglobin in vivo. J. Clin. Invest. 57. In press. 1976.

[9]Bunn, H. F., Haney, D. N., Gabbay, K. H., and Gallop, P. M.: Further identifi-

cation of the nature and linkage of the carbohydrate in hemoglobin A_{Ic}. Biochem. Biophys. Res. Com. 67:103–09, 1975.

[10]Keonig, R. J., and Cerami, A.: Glycosylation of hemoglobin in the diabetic mouse. Fed. Proc. 34:335, 1975.

[11]Gandhi, V. S., and Bleicher, S. J.: "Fast" hemoglobin, diabetes and pregnancy. Diabetes 24 (Suppl. 2):415, 1975.

[12]Osterby, R.: Morphometric studies of the peripheral glomerular basement in early juvenile diabetes mellitus. I. Development of initial basement membrane thickening. Diabetologia 8:84–92, 1972.

[13]Kilo, C., Vogler, N., and Williamson, J. R.: Muscle capillary basement membrane changes related to aging and diabetes mellitus. Diabetes 21:881–905, 1972.

[14]Jackson, R., Guthrie, R., Esterly, J., Bilginturan, N., James, R., Yeast, J., Saathoff, J., and Guthrie, D.: Muscle capillary basement membrane changes in normal and diabetic children. Diabetes 24 (Suppl. 2):400, 1975.

[15]Job, D., Eschwege, E., Guyot, C., and Tchobroutsky, G.: Effect of multiple daily insulin injections on the course of diabetic retinopathy. Diabetes 24 (Suppl. 2):397, 1975.

Appendix E

VALUABLE BASIC AND REFERENCE TEXTS

This manual assumes that the reader already has certain elementary knowledge about diabetes and its treatment—such as how to mix, inject, and store insulin, etc. Newly diagnosed patients (and their families), as well as those who have not had training in depth, can derive considerable benefit from reading at least the first two of the following excellent basic texts. We consider the *Joslin Diabetes Manual* to be essential reading for all diabetics. It should be noted, however, that the GLUCOGRAF method advocates regimens of insulin, diet, and scheduling which differ considerably from the traditional approaches found in the following references.

Food Values of Portions Commonly Used should be of value to anyone interested in the contents of foods. It lists protein, fat, carbohydrate, calories, polyunsaturated fatty acids, vitamins, minerals, and fiber content of about 5,000 foods and is used as a bible by many dietitians.

Any of the four volumes listed below can be ordered through your local bookstore or directly from the publisher.

Joslin Diabetes Manual. 11th ed. Edited by Leo P. Krall, M.D. Philadelphia: Lea & Febiger, 1978.

Diabetes: The New Approach. Milton J. Brothers, M.D. New York: Grosset & Dunlap, 1976.

Managing Diabetics Properly: Nursing Skillbook. Horsham, Pa.: Intermed Communications, 1977.

Food Values of Portions Commonly Used. 13th ed. Edited by J. Pennington and H. Church. Philadelphia: J. B. Lippincott Company, 1980.

Appendix F

INFORMATIVE REFERENCES FROM SCIENTIFIC JOURNALS

This list is intended for possible use by the clinician who does not specialize in the treatment of diabetes and may therefore be unfamiliar with the recent scientific literature in this field. Material abstracted by the popular press and the more general medical journals has tended to concentrate on the more sensational advances, leaving the gradual elucidation of basic mechanisms hidden from view.

The references cited encompass a fraction of 1 percent of the diabetes literature of the past six years. They have been selected for pertinence to the regimen and many of the points discussed in this manual. Most of them contain information that has direct or indirect bearing on approaches to the treatment of diabetes.

References

1. American Dietetic Association. Dietary Goals for the United States, Second Edition, 1977: A Reaction Statement by the American Dietetic Association, *Diabetes Care* 2:278–282 (1979).

2. Anderson, J.; Midgley, W.; and Wedman, B. Fiber and Diabetes, *Diabetes Care* 2:369–379 (1979).

3. Anderson, J.W.; Lin, W.; and Ward, K. Composition of Foods Commonly Used in Diets for Persons with Diabetes, *Diabetes Care* 1:293–302 (1978).

4. Asplin, C.; Hartog, M.; and Goldie, D. Change of Insulin Dosage, Circulating Free and Bound Insulin and Insulin Antibodies on Transferring Diabetics from Conventional to Highly Purified Porcine Insulin, *Diabetologia* 14:99–106 (1978).

5. Aydin, I.; Raskin, P.; and Unger, R. The Effect of Short-Term Intravenous Insulin Administration on the Glucagon Response to a Carbohydrate Meal in Adult Onset and Juvenile Type Diabetes, *Diabetologia* 13:629–636 (1977).

6. Bernstein, R.K. Virtually Continuous Euglycemia for Five Years in a Labile Juvenile Onset Diabetic Under Non-Invasive Closed-loop Control, *Diabetes Care* 3:140–143 (1980).

7. Bleicher, S., chairman. Symposium on Home Blood Glucose Monitoring, *Diabetes Care* 3:57–186 (1979).

8. ———; Lee, T.; Bernstein, R.; Schacter, L.; Temes, R.; Krupin, T.; Santiago, J.; Becker, B.; and Waltman, S. Effect of Blood Glucose Control on Retinal Vascular Permeability in Insulin-Dependent Diabetes Mellitus, *Diabetes Care* 3:184–186 (1980).

9. Bressler, R., and Galloway, J. The Insulins: Pharmacology and Uses, *Drug Therapy* 8:43–61 (1978).

10. Brownlee, M., and Cahill, G.F. Diabetic Control and Vascular Complications, *Atherosclerosis Review* 4:29–70 (1979).

11. Cahill, G.; Field, J.; and Wiseman, E., eds. Progress Toward Understanding and Treating Diabetic Complications: Proceedings of a Symposium, *Metabolism* 28:387–488 (1979).

12. Christensen, N.J. Catecholamines and Diabetes Mellitus, *Diabetologia* 16:211–224 (1979).

13. Clements, R.S., Jr. Diabetic Neuropathy: New Concepts of Its Etiology, *Diabetes* 28:604–611 (1979).

14. Covinsky, J.; Kelley, K.; and Hamburger, S. Hormonal Relationships of the Endocrine Pancreas in Diabetes Mellitus, *J. Amer. Women's Med. Assoc.* 34:12–20 (1979).

15. Crapo, P.; Reaven, G.; and Olefsky, J. Postprandial Plasma–Glucose and Insulin Responses to Different Complex Carbohydrates, *Diabetes* 26:1178–1183 (1977).

16. Cunha-Vaz, J.; Fonseca, J.; Abreu, J.; and Ruas, M. Detection of Early Retinal Changes by Vitreous Fluorophotometry, *Diabetes* 28:16–19 (1979).

17. Deckert, T. Intermediate-acting Insulin Preparations, *Diabetes Care* 3:623–626 (1980).

18. ———; Poulsen, J.; and Larsen, M. Prognosis of Diabetics with Diabetes Onset Before the Age of Thirty-one. II: Factors Influencing the Prognosis, *Diabetologia* 14:371–378 (1978).

19. Dunbar, J.C.; Walsh, M.F.; and Foa, P.P. The Serum Glucose Response to Glucagon Suppression with Somatostatin, Insulin, or Antiglucagon Serum in Depancreatized Rats, *Diabetologia* 14:53–58 (1978).

20. Dupuis, A.; Jones, R.; and Peterson, C. Diabetes: Psychological Effects of Glucose Self-Monitoring, *Psychosomatics* 21:581–591 (1980).

21. Eaton, R.P. Lipids and Diabetes: The Case for Treatment of Microvascular Disease (review article), *Diabetes Care* 2:46–50 (1979).

22. ———, *et al.* Diabetic Glucose Control: Matching Plasma Insulin Concentration to Dietary and Stress Hyperglycemia, *Diabetes Care* 1:40–44 (1978).

23. Engerman. R.; Bloodworth, J.; and Nelson, S. Relationship of Microvascular Disease in Diabetes to Metabolic Control, *Diabetes* 26:760–769 (1977).

24. Felig, P.; Wahren, J.; Sherwin, R.; and Hendler, R. Insulin, Glucagon, and Somatostatin in Normal Physiology and Diabetes Mellitus (Lilly Lecture, 1976), *Diabetes* 25:1091–1099 (1976).

25. Gale, E.; Kurtz, A.; and Tattersall, R. The Myth of Rebound Hypoglycemia, *Diabetes* 28:349 (1979).

26. Galloway, J. A. Insulin Treatment for the Early 80's: Facts and Questions About Old and New Insulins and Their Usage, *Diabetes Care* 3:615–622 (1980).

27. ———, *et al.* The Bioavailability of Regular Insulin in Normal Fasted Subjects—The Effect of Mixing with NPH and Lente, of Depth and of Method of Administration, *Diabetes* 28:355 (1979).

28. Ganda, O.P. Pathogenesis of Macrovascular Disease in the Human Diabetic (review article), *Diabetes* 29:931–942 (1980).

29. Genuth, S.M. Plasma Insulin and Glucose Profiles in Normal, Obese, and Diabetic Persons, *Annals of Internal Medicine* 79:812–822 (1973).

30. Gonen, B., and Rubenstein, A. Haemoglobin A_1 and Diabetes Mellitus, *Diabetologia* 15:1–8 (1978).

31. Goodkin, G. Mortality Factors in Diabetes, *Journal of Occupational Medicine* 17:716–721 (1975).

32. Goulder, T., and Alberti, K. Dietary Fibre and Diabetes (editorial), *Diabetologia* 15:285–287 (1978).

33. Graf, R., *et al.* Motor Nerve Conduction Velocity in Untreated Diabetics: A Function of Levels of Hyperglycemia, *Diabetes* 27 (Supplement 2):435 (1978).

34. Grundy, S. High Density Lipoprotein and Atherosclerosis, *Resident and Staff Physician* (February 1980): 3s–18s.

35. Hamburger, S. Diabetic Ketoacidosis, *Journal of American Women's Medical Association* 34:109–127 (1979).

36. Hedtmann, A., and Gruneklee, D. C-Peptide Determination in Urine, a Useful Index for Estimation of Pancreatic B-Cell Function. *Diabetologia* 15:238 (1978).

37. Hepp, K.D. Studies on the Mechanism of Insulin Action: Basic Concepts and Clinical Implications (review article), *Diabetologia* 13:177–186 (1977).

38. Herbert, V. MegaVitamin Therapy. *New York State Journal of Medicine* (February 1979):278–279.

39. Horwitz, D.L.; Rubenstein, A.H.; and Katz, A.I. Quantitation of Human Pancreatic Beta-Cell Function by Immunoassay of C-Peptide in Urine, *Diabetes* 26:30–35 (1977).

40. Hulst, S.G. Th. Treatment of Insulin Induced Lipoatrophy, *Diabetes* 25:1052–1054 (1976).

41. Jackson, R., *et al.* Development of Microvascular Changes in Children and Young Adults with Insulin Dependent Diabetes, *Diabetes* 28:409 (1979).

42. Jeanrenaud, B. Insulin and Obesity, *Diabetologia* 17:133–138 (1979).

43. Kahn, C., and Rosenthal, A. Immunologic Reactions to Insulin: Insulin Allergy, Insulin Resistance, and the Autoimmune Syndrome (review), *Diabetes Care* 2:283–295 (1979).

44. Kalkhoff, R., and Levin, M. The Saccharine Controversy, *Diabetes Care* 1:211–222 (1978).

45. Koivusto, V. Variations in Glycemic Control and Insulin Absorption Rates from Different Injection Sites in Diabetic Subjects, *Diabetes* 28:355 (1979).

46. Krupin, T., *et al.* Vitreous Fluorophotometry in Juvenile Onset Diabetes Mellitus. *Arch. Ophthal.* 96:812–814 (1978).

47. Kuebler, T., *et al.* Abnormalities of Nerve Conduction Time in Diabetes Are Correlated with Hyperglycemia but Not Duration of Disease, *Diabetes* 28:415 (1979).

48. Lopes-Virella, M., and Woltmann, H. Plasma High Density Lipoprotein Cholesterol Increases with Control in Insulin-Dependent Young Male Diabetics, *Diabetes* 28:348 (1979).

49. ———, *et al.* Early Diagnosis of Renal Malfunction in Diabetics, *Diabetologia* 16:165–172 (1979).

50. Luft, R.; Efendic, S.; and Hokfelt, T. Somatostatin—Both Hormone and Neurotransmitter, *Diabetologia* 14:1–14 (1978).

51. McMillan, D., and Ditzel, J., eds. Journal of Proceedings of a Conference on Diabetic Microangiopathy, *Diabetes* 25:805–930 (1976).

52. McNair, P., *et al.* Influence of Metabolic Control on Osteopenia in Insulin Treated Diabetes, *Diabetologia* 15:254 (1978).

53. Nabarro, J., *et al.* Insulin Deficient Diabetes (review article), *Diabetologia* 16:5–12 (1979).

54. National Diabetes Data Group. Classification and Diagnosis of Diabetes Mellitus and Other Categories of Glucose Intolerance, *Diabetes* 28:1039–1057 (1979).

55. Peterson, C., *et al.* Reversible Hematologic Sequelae of Diabetes Mellitus, *Annals of Internal Medicine* 86:425–429 (1977).

56. ———; Jones, R.; Dupuis, A.; Levine, B.; Bernstein, R.; and O'Shea, M. Feasibility of Improved Blood Glucose Con-

trol in Patients with Insulin Dependent Diabetes Mellitus, *Diabetes Care* 2:329–335 (1979).

57. ——, *et al.* Changes in Basement Membrane Thickening and Pulse Volume Concomitant with Improved Glucose Control and Exercise in Patients with Insulin-Dependent Diabetes Mellitus, *Diabetes Care* 3:586–589 (1980).

58. Pirart, J. Diabetes Mellitus and Its Degenerative Complications: A Prospective Study of 4400 Patients Observed Between 1947 and 1973, *Diabete et Metabolisme* 3:97–107; 173–182, 245–256 (1977); and *Diabetes Care* 1:168–188, 252–263 (1978).

59. Radhakrishnamurthy, B., *et al.* Serum-Free and Protein-Bound Sugars and Cardiovascular Complications in Diabetes Mellitus, *Laboratory Investigation* 34:159–165 (1976).

60. Rasch, R. Prevention of Diabetic Glomerulopathy by Careful Insulin Treatment: Experimental Studies of the Mesangial Regions, *Diabetologia* 15:264 (1978).

61. Reaven, G.; Sageman, W.; and Swenson, R. Development of Insulin Resistance in Normal Dogs Following Alloxan-Induced Deficiency, *Diabetologia* 13:459–462 (1977).

62. Reinila, A., and Akerblom, H. Accumulation of Lipids in the Pulmonary Artery of Diabetic Rats and the Effect of Insulin Treatment, *Diabetologia* 15:265 (1978).

63. Sestoft, L. Fructose and the Dietary Therapy of Diabetes Mellitus (editorial), *Diabetologia* 17:1–4 (1979).

64. Sherwin, R., and Felig, P. Pathophysiology of Diabetes Mellitus, *Medical Clinics of North America* 62:695–711 (1978).

65. Siegel, E.; Trapp, V.; and Schmidt, F. Response of Parameters of Carbohydrate and Lipid Metabolism in 10-

Month Diabetic Rats to Extreme Reduction of the Carbohydrate Supply in the Food, *Diabetologia* 12:419 (1976).

66. ———. Effect of CHO Restriction on Pancreatic Insulin and Severity of Long-Term Diabetes in Rats, *Diabetes* 27:504 (1978).

67. Simonds, J.F. Psychiatric Status of Diabetic Youth in Good and Poor Control, *International Journal of Psychiatry in Medicine* 7:133–151 (1976).

68. ———. Psychiatric Status of Diabetic Youth Matched with a Control Group, *Diabetes* 26:921–925 (1977).

69. Skyler, J.S. Complications of Diabetes Mellitus: Relationship to Metabolic Dysfunction, *Diabetes Care* 2:499–509 (1979).

70. ———. Diabetes and Exercise: Clinical Implications, *Diabetes Care* 2:307–311 (1979).

71. ———. A Plethora of Insulins, *Diabetes Care* 3:638–639 (1980).

72. Sosenko, J., *et al.* Relationship between Lipid and Glucose Fluctuations in Young Insulin Dependent Diabetics, *Diabetes* 28:415 (1979).

73. Spiro, R.G. Search for a Biochemical Basis of Diabetic Microangiopathy (review article), *Diabetologia* 12:1–14 (1976).

74. Steiner, D.F. On the Role of the Proinsulin C-peptide, in: Proceedings of an International C-peptide Research Symposium, *Diabetes* 27:145–285 (1978).

75. Sullivan, Barbara-Jean. Self-esteem and Depression in Adolescent Diabetic Girls, *Diabetes Care* 1:18–19 (1978).

76. Takeshi, K., *et al.* C-peptide Immunoreactivity (CPR) in Urine, *Diabetes* 27:210–215 (1978).

77. Tchobroutsky, G. Relation of Diabetic Control to Devel-

opment of Microvascular Complications, *Diabetologia* 15: 143–152 (1978).

78. Trapp, V., *et al.* Long Term Study of the Effects of Extremely Low Carbohydrate Diets on Diabetes-Induced Late Changes in the Lens, Retina, Nerve, and Kidneys of Rats, *Diabetologia* 12:423 (1976).

79. Unger, R., and Orci, L. Possible Roles of the Pancreatic D-Cell in the Normal and Diabetic States, *Diabetes* 26:241–244 (1977).

80. Viberti, G.C., *et al.* Effect of Control of Blood Glucose on Urinary Excretion of Albumin and B_2 Microglobulin in Insulin-Dependent Diabetes, *New England Journal of Medicine* 300:638–641 (1979).

81. *Journal of Visual Impairment and Blindness* 72:337–384 (1978) (entire issue is devoted to diabetes).

82. Vranic, M., and Berger, M. Exercise and Diabetes Mellitus, *Diabetes* 28:147–167 (1979).

83. Vranic, M.; Horvath, S.; and Warren, J, eds. Proceedings of a Conference on Diabetes and Exercise, *Diabetes* 28:1–113 (1979).

84. Waltman, S.; Oestrich, C.; Krupin, T.; Hanish, S.; Ratzan, S.; Santiago, J.; and Kilo, C. Quantitative Vitreous Fluorophotometry, *Diabetes* 27:85–87 (1978).

85. Witztum, J., and Schonfeld, G. High Density Lipoproteins (review and abstracts), *Diabetes* 28:326–336 (1979).

86. Wolinsky, H. A New Look at Atherosclerosis, *Cardiovascular Medicine* (September 1976):41–54.

87. Wunschell, I., and Sheikolislam, B. Is There a Role for Dietetic Foods in the Management of Diabetes and/or Obesity? *Diabetes Care* 1:247–249 (1978).

88. Yue, D., and Turtle, J. New Forms of Insulin and Their Use in the Treatment of Diabetes, *Diabetes* 26:341–347 (1977).

Appendix G

FOR USERS OF THE DISCONTINUED EYETONE REFLECTANCE COLORIMETER

Reprinted from
Diabetes Care 2, no. 2 (March-April 1979)
Copyright 1979 by the American Diabetes Association, Inc.

Blood Glucose Self-Monitoring by Diabetic Patients: Refinements of Procedural Technique

RICHARD K. BERNSTEIN

A number of groups[1-6] have recently reported their experiences with the use of home blood glucose monitoring as an aid to achievement of improved diabetic control. Most of these groups have used the Dextrostix/Eyetone System (Ames Company, Elkhart, Indiana). This system entails the use of a glucose oxidase-impregnated reagent strip (Dextrostix), which on exposure to blood undergoes a colorimetric reaction proportional to blood glucose concentration. The Eyetone reflectance colorimeter allows for convenient quantitation of the reaction. The author, an engineer with insulin-dependent diabetes mellitus, has used this system for home blood glucose monitoring since 1971, having made more than 15,000 determinations in that time span. Observations from this experience have led to refinements of the procedural techniques that allow for improved utility of the system. Many of these refinements have been used by clinicians and patients who employ the Dextrostix/Eyetone System for home blood glucose monitoring. In view of the growing use of such monitoring, these procedural refine-ments

are outlined here. They fall into three broad categories: (1) finger puncture; (2) handling of reagent strips; and (3) meter operation.

FINGER PUNCTURE

1. Free flow of blood can be enhanced, especially in cold weather, by holding the hand under warm, running tap water, prior to puncture, for about 20 s. (Caution must be exerted not to use hot water, particularly if neuropathy is present.)

2. Although any finger may be selected as a source of blood, the thumb seems to serve this function better than the other digits, because of its greater surface area and superior blood supply. (The dual blood supply of the fourth finger makes this a better choice than the remaining fingers.)

3. Disposable lancets formed from wire, of round cross section, are preferred over lancets stamped from sheet metal because the latter produce a more painful wound that heals less rapidly. Hypodermic needles of gauges 27, 28, or 29 can serve as satisfactory lancets with the smaller gauges preferred. Disposable needles may be reused about 12 times without losing much

---

1. Reference numbers apply to references at the end of this appendix.

sharpness. They should, however, be wiped with an alcohol sponge before and after use and stored in a closed container if they are to be reused.

The Monolet lancet (Sherwood Medical Industries, Deland, Florida), while not as sharp as the aforementioned hypodermic needles, is also of round cross section and offers the advantages of low cost (about 3¢ each) and a plastic handle that prevents penetration beyond a depth of 3 mm.

4. The ball of the finger is usually a more painful puncture site than the *peripheral* palmar surface of the distal phalanx. This less painful surface is "U" shaped and begins just above the distal joint, continuing around the periphery of the tip and back towards the same joint on the opposite side of the finger (Figure 1).

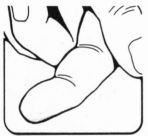

FIG. 1. *Peripheral palmar surface of distal phalanx (shaded) is usually a less painful puncture site than ball of finger.*

5. Pain can be reduced if the patient presses the target digit with an opposing digit of the same hand while the puncture is being made (Figure 2). Pressure should be applied to the palmar surface immediately above the distal joint and should be

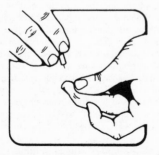

FIG. 2. *Pressure from opposing digit can reduce pain of puncture.*

great enough to cause a marked erythema of the distal phalanx.

6. Before stabbing, the finger must be dry. Any surface moisture will cause blood to spread over the surface instead of accumulating in a compact drop that can be easily transferred to the reagent strip.

METER OPERATION

7. It is not necessary to wipe off the first drop of blood as recommended in some clinical laboratory manuals. Results appear to be unaffected by this extra step.

8. A proper wound will rapidly produce a drop of blood at least 5 mm in diameter without prolonged "milking" of the finger. If free flow is not obtained, wipe off the finger and puncture again. This will prevent dilution of the specimen with tissue fluid.

HANDLING OF REAGENT STRIPS

1. A plastic squeeze bottle, similar to that supplied by the manufacturer of the reagent strips, should be used to wash blood from the reagent strip. Running tap water does not usually have adequate velocity for rapid, complete removal of blood.

2. When washing blood from the strip, the untreated side should rest against the vertical inside surface of a tumbler or sink, so that it is restrained from flopping back and forth in the stream of water (Figure 3).

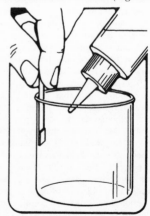

FIG. 3. *Untreated side of reagent strip should rest against vertical inside surface of tumbler or sink while washing off blood.*

3. After color development, washing and blotting, the treated surface of the strip should be uniform in color. Blotches or mottling indicate improper technique and incorrect results.

1. The principle cause of grossly false blood glucose measurement by patients is their failure to recalibrate the meter prior to each use. The calibration procedure set forth in the Eyetone instruction manual is designed for the clinical laboratory, not for the patient. The procedure assumes that a batch of blood glucoses is being processed in sequence. It therefore calls for the use of a gravimetrically prepared solution (Dextrostix Calibration and Control Set, Ames Company, Elkhart, Indiana) containing 130 mg/dl of glucose, prior to each batch of blood glucose determinations. When this procedure is followed by a patient, an additional Dextrostix must be used for every blood glucose measurement, thus doubling the cost. As a result, patients rarely observe the procedure, and most measurements are erroneous.

The following method uses a secondary standard to replace the extra Dextrostix and the glucose solution, while still compensating for differences between batches of reagent strips and differences in technique from one operator to another.

(a) Once every month, recheck the high and low calibration points using the "Set 1" and "Set 2" gray strips and following the procedure set forth by the manufacturer. These settings will remain stable for long periods if the "Set 1" and "Set 2" control knobs are not rotated after the initial adjustment.

(b) A newly opened vial of reagent strips must be calibrated against both a glucose standard and a secondary standard. The secondary standard will be the "Set 2" gray strip. First a drop of glucose solution of known concentration (e.g. 130 mg/dl vial from the Dextrostix Calibration and Control Set) is placed on a reagent strip, and color is developed in the usual manner. The developed strip is inserted in the meter and the instrument is adjusted (by rotating the black knurled wheel) until a reading equal to the known glucose concentration (in this example, 130 mg/dl) appears. The meter is now calibrated for the new vial of reagent strips. This calibration, however, may drift from day to day or from use to use. To preserve this calibration, immediately remove the used reagent strip and insert the "Set 2" gray strip. Secure a meter reading on the gray strip, and write this value and the calibration date, on the label of the new vial of reagent strips. (Recent batches of Dextrostix have been giving readings of 65 mg/dl on the "Set 2" strip when the 130 mg/dl glucose standard is used.) The "Set 2" gray strip together with the number written on the vial serves as a secondary standard for future blood glucose measurements using this vial of reagent strips.

(c) When performing a blood glucose measurement, the procedure is very simple. Immediately after applying blood to a reagent strip (i.e. while the strip is developing), turn on the meter and wait 20 seconds for the filament brightness to stabilize. Insert the "Set 2" gray strip and adjust the instrument (black knurled wheel) so that the meter reading is identical to the number previously written on the vial. This operation requires perhaps another 20 seconds and can be completed before the blood is washed from the reagent strip. Next, remove the gray strip from the meter, wash off and blot the reagent strip, and insert it into the instrument. Immediately read BG.

2. There is a tendency for patients to accidently discard the "Set 2" gray strips that play such an important role in calibration. This is especially frequent during periods of hypoglycemia. It is, therefore, advisable that the "Set 2" strip be taped to the instrument in such a way that the proper end can be conveniently inserted and removed from the reading slot (Figure 4). If the plastic strip cracks, at the loop shown in Figure 4, it can be reinforced with cellophane tape.

3. The instruction manual designates a ½ hour warm-up period before the instrument should be used. This requirement is

270

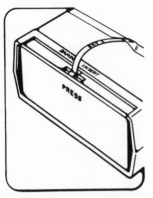

FIG. 4. "Set 2" gray calibration strip, taped to meter to reduce likelihood of loss when used frequently.

based on the fact that there is a slight drift in instrument response, perhaps 1 mg/dl per minute after it is first turned on. This requirement is necessary only for clinical laboratory use, where a batch of blood glucose measurements are being made and where there may be a long delay between calibration and reading the last blood glucose of the batch. Warm-up is totally unnecessary for patient use, where the delay between calibration and reading blood glucose is less than 1 minute. This unnecessary requirement has discouraged many patients from carrying meters with them when away from home, because they feel that they will not have time to wait for the instrument to stabilize.

4. If blood glucose measurements are performed less frequently than twice daily, the reagent strips in a vial of 100 pieces will last longer than one month. In such cases, it is wise to recalibrate the vial every month to prevent errors resulting from reduced enzyme activity in the sensitive region of the strips. It is, therefore, advisable for the patient to write on every vial the date of each calibration.

5. If the patient observes the developed color of each strip prior to inserting it in the meter, he will probably, in time, develop a skill at reading strips by eye—especially for blood glucose levels in or near the normal range. This skill diminishes if the patient fails to use the meter regularly. If an instrument is disabled or if the patient cannot always carry the meter with him, he

can resort to visual readings. The author can usually read a strip with an accuracy of ±5 mg/dl over the range 50–180 mg/dl.

6. The Eyetone manufacturer has provided salesmen with extra colorimeters that can be loaned to patients while their instruments are being repaired. Patients should phone their local representative or the company medical director to secure this emergency service.

7. The plastic wash bottle supplied with the Eyetone instrument is not easy to replace and is occasionally left by patients in public washrooms, etc.; therefore, it is wise for the patient to request several extra bottles when purchasing a meter. The prescribing physician or clinic might also wish to keep extra bottles on hand as a service to patients.

8. Several manufacturers are developing small, battery-operated meters for patient use. Some forthcoming meters may store their secondary glucose standard in a microcircuit program that the operator can adjust. These may or may not be designed around calibration strips, such as the "Set 1" and "Set 2" gray strips used with the Eyetone where a permanently colored strip may be of value as a secondary glucose standard, it might become necessary for physicians or clinics to fabricate their own. This may be done readily, by using a permanent-type, light color, felt-tip marker to darken the sensitive area of an unused reagent strip. The depth of color should be such that, when another reagent strip is read after exposure to a known glucose solution (within normal blood glucose range), the secondary standard will give a meter reading within ±50% of the glucose solution reading.

<hr />

CONCLUSION

Self-monitoring of blood glucose by insulin-dependent diabetic patients has become increasingly prevalent, particularly in view of the growing evidence of the value of maintaining euglycemia.[7-9] Manufacturers of systems for rapid blood glucose measurement, using capillary blood and reagent strips, have not yet oriented instrument manuals toward patient needs. This report should aid clinicians and patients in refining the techniques of self-monitoring in an effort to improve the accuracy of the measurement process.

R. K. Bernstein is a guest collaborator at The Rockefeller University, New York, and a research associate at Brooklyn Hospital, Brooklyn, New York.

REFERENCES

[1]Danowski, T. S., and Sunder, J. H.: Jet injection of insulin during self-monitoring of blood glucose. Diabetes Care 1: 27–33, 1978.

[2]Skyler, J. S., Lasky, I. A., Skyler, D. L., Robertson, E. G., and Mintz, D. H.: Home blood glucose monitoring as an aid in diabetes management. Diabetes Care 1: 150–157, 1978.

[3]Sonksen, P. H., Judd, S. L., and Lowy, C.: Home monitoring of blood glucose—method for improving diabetic control. Lancet 1: 729–732, 1978.

[4]Walford, S., Gale, E. A. M., Allison, S. P., and Tattersall, R. B.: Self-monitoring of blood glucose—improvement of diabetic control. Lancet 1: 732–735, 1978.

[5]Peterson, C. M., Jones, R. L., Dupuis, A., Bernstein, R., and O'Shea, M.: Feasibility of tight control of juvenile diabetes through patient-monitored glucose determinations. Diabetes 27 (Suppl. 2): 437, 1978.

[6]Ikeda, Y., Tajima, N., Minami, N., Ide, Y., Yokoyama, J., and Abe, M.: Pilot study of self-measurement of blood glucose using the Dextrostix-Eyetone system for juvenile-onset diabetes. Diabetologia 15: 91–93, 1978.

[7]Pirart, J.: Diabetes mellitus and its degenerative complications: a prospective study of 4,400 patients observed between 1947 and 1973. Diabete et Metabolisme 3: 97–107, 173–182, 245–256, 1977; and Diabetes Care 1: 168–188, 252–263, 1978.

[8]Skyler, J. S.: "Control" and complications. Editorial. Diabetes Care 1: 204–205, 1978.

[9]Brownlee, M., and Cahill, G. F.: Diabetic control and vascular complications. Atherosclerosis Rev. 4: 29–70, 1979.

Appendix H

FOREIGN EQUIVALENTS OF INSULINS
AVAILABLE IN THE U.S.

Some of the foreign brands are available only as pork or as single-component insulins, and may, therefore, be effective for some patients in lower doses than the American mixed beef/pork equivalents.

Insulin Action	U.S. Designation (Manufacturer)	Foreign Equivalents
Rapid	Regular (Lilly, Squibb) Velosulin [1] (Nordisk) Actrapid [1] (Novo)	Neutral, Toronto, Actrapid, Insular, Insulina, Insulina Simple, Neusulin, Insuline, Insuline Simple, Insulyl, Insulin, Insulin Quick, Crystalline, Soluble
	Semilente (Lilly, Squibb) Semitard [1] (Novo)	Semitard, Demi-Dura, Semilente, Semilenta, Subtardum
Intermediate	NPH (Lilly, Squibb) Insulatard [1] (Nordisk)	Isophane, Rapitard, Retard, Protard, Neuphane
	Mixtard [1] (Nordisk)	Mixtard
	Lente (Lilly, Squibb) Lentard (Novo) Monotard [1] (Novo)	Monotard, Lentard, Dura, Lenta, Lente, Lente Zinc, Tardum, Neulente

1. Only available as pure pork insulin.

Prolonged	Ultralente (Lilly, Squibb) Ultratard (Novo)	Ultratard, Ultralente, Extra-dura, Extra Tardum
	Protamine Zinc (Lilly, Squibb)	Protamine Zinc, Depotinsulin, Depotinsulyl, Depsulin, Insulyl Retard, Endopancrine Zinc-protamine

Appendix I

GLOSSARY

A-cells Specialized endocrine cells, located in the islets of Langerhans of the pancreas, which manufacture glucagon and release it into the bloodstream. Also called Alpha cells.

Adipose Fatty, fat.

Amino acids The molecular building blocks of proteins.

Antibodies Protein produced by the body in response to the presence of foreign cells or molecules, such as animal insulins, viruses, bacteria, toxins, etc. Antibodies attach permanently or temporarily to the foreign material, rendering it inactive.

ATP Adenosine triphosphate. A chemical used by the body to transfer energy derived from foodstuffs to various forms of work such as muscular activity, transport of substances into and out of cells, etc.

B-cells Specialized endocrine cells, located in the islets of Langerhans of the pancreas, which manufacture insulin and release it into the bloodstream. Also called Beta cells.

Basal insulin requirement The insulin required to maintain normal body glucose (BG) levels in a person who is fasting and not physically active. In the regimen described in this manual, usually provided by Ultralente insulin.

BG Blood glucose concentration. Nondiabetics usually have fasting values in the range 70–120 milligrams per deciliter (mg/dl).

274

Binding sites See *Receptor sites.*

Blood glucose Blood sugar. Elevated in untreated diabetes. The principal fuel for most cells of the body.

Bread exchange A food portion containing 12 grams of carbohydrate (CHO), the same amount as in one standard slice of bread.

Brittle diabetes A type of diabetes, usually characterized by little or no production of endogenous insulin, in which small feedings of carbohydrate or protein will cause great increases in BG. Improper treatment of this form of diabetes usually results in extreme daily BG swings between very low and very high values. Also called "juvenile" diabetes, "juvenile-onset" diabetes, "insulin-dependent" diabetes (IDDM), and in this manual "Type Ia" diabetes.

Capillary blood Blood removed from microscopic vessels such as those near the surface of the skin—for example, finger-puncture blood.

Carbohydrate Sugars or complexes formed by the conjunction of two or more sugar molecules. The principal source of dietary energy (calories) in the diets of most "advanced" countries. Also includes monosaccharides.

Cardiovascular Relating to the heart (cardio) and blood vessels (vascular), arteries in particular.

Catecholamines The endocrine hormones adrenalin (also called epinephrine) and noradrenalin (norepinephrine). Produced in the adrenal medulla and also in nerve tissue where they act as neurotransmitters. They serve several counter-regulatory functions in glucose metabolism, such as breakdown of muscle and liver glycogen to glucose and inhibition of insulin release from the pancreatic B-cell. They also facilitate the breakdown of fatty acids as an alternate source of fuel.

CHO   Abbreviation for carbohydrate.

Cholesterol   A lipid that is continually manufactured and destroyed in the body. In poorly controlled diabetes and in cardiovascular diseases, blood levels are frequently high. Cholesterol deposited inside blood vessels is believed to be a major causative factor in cardiovascular disease.

Complex sugars   Polysaccharides. Large carbohydrate molecules consisting of many simple-sugar building blocks joined together. Digested more slowly than simple sugars. Also called "complex carbohydrates."

Counter-regulatory hormones   Hormones that oppose the action of insulin by raising BG and breaking down glycogen, body fats, and proteins. These hormones include glucagon, glucocorticoids, catecholamines, and growth hormone.

C-peptide   A chain of amino acids (a peptide) that connects the A and B chains of the proinsulin molecule. (See Fig. 1.) The pancreatic B-cell releases C-peptide into the bloodstream when insulin is formed from proinsulin. The presence of C-peptide in the blood or urine is evidence that endogenous insulin is being produced. Higher C-peptide levels indicate greater rates of insulin output. Also called "connecting peptide."

Dextrose   Glucose.

Diabetes mellitus   A disease characterized by inability to fully utilize glucose as a source of energy. Commonly called "diabetes."

Disaccharide   A carbohydrate built from the linkage of 2 sugar molecules. Examples include sucrose (glucose + fructose), lactose (glucose + galactose) and maltose (glucose + glucose).

Endocrine glands   Glands containing tissues that release hormones directly into the bloodstream: thyroid, pancreas, adrenal, pituitary, others.

Endogenous   Produced within the organism. Insulin secreted by the pancreas is endogenous insulin. See *Exogenous*.

Euglycemia   The state of having blood glucose within the normal range.

Exogenous   Originating outside the organism. Exogenous insulin is injected insulin.

Glucagon   An endocrine hormone produced by the A-cells of the pancreas and by cells in the intestines. Opposes the action of insulin, in that it signals the liver to break down stored fuels, converting them to rapidly available energy sources. It causes BG to increase because certain stored fuels are convertible to glucose.

Glucocorticoids   Counter-regulatory hormones secreted by the adrenal cortex: cortisone, corticosterone, hydrocortisone, etc.

Gluconeogenesis   The process by which amino acids are converted to glucose in the liver.

Glucose   A simple sugar, present in blood and other tissues, which serves as the major source of immediate fuel for the cells of the body. Also called dextrose and D-glucose.

Glucose tolerance   The ability of an organism to lower its own BG after BG has been elevated by ingestion of carbohydrate or by intravenous injection of certain sugars. This ability is impaired in diabetes.

Glycogen   A starchlike polysaccharide, consisting of interconnected chains of glucose molecules. Stored in liver and muscles as a reserve source of fuel. Can be broken down to glucose in the presence of certain counter-regulatory hormones.

Glycogenesis   The process whereby glycogen reserves are created from glucose.

Glycogenolysis   The process by which liver and muscles break glycogen down to glucose.

Glycosylated hemoglobin   Hemoglobin to which one or more glucose molecules have been attached. Elevated levels are found in poorly controlled diabetes. Concentration reflects average control of BG over prior 1–3 weeks. See HbA_1 and HbA_{1c}.

HbA_1   The total of glycosylated hemoglobins in the blood. $HbA_{1a1} + HbA_{1a2} + HbA_{1b} + HbA_{1c}$.

HbA_{1c}   A particular glycosylated hemoglobin that is especially sensitive to changes in BG.

HDL   High-density lipoprotein. More properly called HDL cholesterol. That portion of total cholesterol carried in the blood by high-density lipoproteins. High serum levels of this particular cholesterol fraction correlate with reduced risk of cardiovascular disease. Blood levels of HDL are frequently raised by physical exercise and may be lowered by uncontrolled diabetes.

Hemoglobin   The red pigment, present in red blood cells, that transports oxygen from the lungs to the various tissues of the body.

Hormones   Chemical messengers that are released into the bloodstream and regulate a variety of processes at various locations in the body, which may be quite distant from the source of the hormone.

Hyperglycemia Elevation of BG above the normal nondiabetic range for a given age and state of feeding. High BG.

Hypoglycemia Low BG, insulin "reaction," insulin "shock." May occur with or without gross clinical symptoms.

IBW Ideal body weight.

IDDM Insulin-dependent diabetes mellitus. Type I diabetes.

Insulin The hormone secreted by the B-cells of the pancreas. Required by most tissues in order to utilize glucose. Essential for most anabolic (tissue-building) metabolism. Opposes the release of glucagon from pancreatic A-cells and opposes the catabolic (tissue-destroying) effects of certain counter-regulatory hormones.

Insulin-dependent diabetes Extreme glucose intolerance, requiring daily administration of exogenous (injected) insulin for survival of patient. Ketoacidosis-prone diabetes. Type I diabetes. Onset is frequently prior to age 40.

Insulinopenia Too little insulin in the blood and tissues.

Intestine The digestive tube passing from the stomach to the anus. Divided primarily into the small intestine (upper) and the large intestine (lower). Most nutrients are absorbed through the walls of the small intestine. The large intestine absorbs water from feces, adds certain mineral salts, etc.

Islets of Langerhans Clusters of cells scattered about the tissue of the pancreas that secrete endocrine hormones. The cells in these clusters of islets include B-cells (insulin) and A-cells (glucagon).

Juvenile-onset diabetes Diabetes with onset prior to physiological maturity. Usually brittle, ketoacidosis-prone and insulin-dependent. Accounts for most Type Ia patients.

Ketoacidosis An acute metabolic state that can occur in diabetes when blood levels of insulin are inadequate. Toxic ketonic acids accumulate in blood, ketones appear in urine, and patient becomes dehydrated. If untreated, can result in coma and death.

Ketone Toxic products produced in the liver from fats if glucose cannot enter cells, as when insulin levels are inadequate.

Ketosis A condition characterized by production and buildup of ketones in the body. A less threatening condition than ketoacidosis because the blood is not acidic.

Kidneys Two organs, located above the small of the back, that filter blood—concentrating excesses of certain substances and releasing them, with water, as urine.

L Lente insulin; abbreviation used in this manual. A turbid, intermediate-acting insulin without modifying proteins.

Lipids Substances related to fats with the properties of being nonsoluble or slightly soluble in water, but highly soluble in "nonpolar" solvents like chloroform and ether. Usually found in the blood bound to protein carriers thus forming lipoproteins. High blood levels of certain lipids, such as VLDL cholesterol and triglycerides are probably major risk factors for cardiovascular diseases. Blood levels of high risk lipids are frequently elevated in diabetics during extended periods of frequent high BG levels.

Lipolysis The chemical breakdown of fats into fatty acids and glycerol.

Lipoproteins Molecules consisting of a lipid joined to a protein.

mg/dl Milligrams per deciliter. A unit of concentration.

One mg/dl equals 1/100 gram per liter. A liter is about equal in volume to one quart.

Microangiopathy   A small blood vessel disease that appears in poorly controlled diabetes, characterized by such features as microaneurisms (ballooning), thickening of basement membrane, and leakage of proteins.

mmol/L   Millimoles per liter. A unit of concentration. One mmol/L of glucose = 18 mg/dl. Used in the United Kingdom for reporting blood glucose levels.

Monosaccharide   A simple carbohydrate where every molecule is a simple sugar molecule such as glucose or fructose.

N   NPH insulin; abbreviation used in this manual. Also called isophane insulin. A turbid, intermediate-acting insulin that contains the modifying protein—protamine.

Neuropathy   A loss of myelin coating from peripheral nerves that commonly occurs in poorly controlled diabetes. Symptoms vary depending upon which nerves are involved but include numbness or pain in the feet, impotence, impaired urinary control, etc.

NIDDM   Non-insulin-dependent diabetes mellitus. Type II diabetes.

Nonlinear response to insulin   The lessening effect of insulin upon BG, as BG increases.

Obese   Too heavy, having a body weight 20 percent or more above ideal body weight for height, sex, and build.

Oligosaccharides   Carbohydrates consisting of 2–10 sugar units linked together. Digested more rapidly than polysaccharides but more slowly than simple sugars.

P   Protamine Zinc insulin; abbreviation used in this manual. Also called PZI. A turbid, long-acting insulin that contains the modifying protein—protamine.

Pancreas   A large glandular abdominal organ that secretes digestive enzymes into the intestine and secretes the hormones insulin, gastrin, glucagon, somatastatin, and pancreatic polypeptide into the bloodstream.

Pancreatic   Relating to, or produced by, the pancreas.

Peptide   A molecule consisting of a sequence of amino acids joined end to end, that is not long enough to be considered a protein.

Polysaccharides   Carbohydrates consisting of more than 10 sugar units linked together. Also called complex sugars. More slowly digested than simple sugars and oligosaccharides.

Polyunsaturated fats   Fats that are liquid at body temperature and believed by some authorities to protect against atherosclerosis when included in the diet.

Postprandial   After eating.

Preprandial   Before eating.

Proinsulin   Large precursor of the insulin molecule. Converted to insulin by removal of C-peptide.

Protein   Large molecules, consisting of chains of amino acids, that serve as structural and functional elements of the body and as sources of genetic information. More than 50 percent of the dry weight of animals is protein. Dietary sources include meat, fish, eggs, milk products, and certain plants.

P/S ratio   Dietary ratio between calories from polyunsaturated fats to calories from saturated fats. High P/S ratios may offer protection from certain cardiovascular diseases.

Quantitative vitreous fluorophotometry   A new, very sensitive test for early degeneration of small blood vessels (microangiopathy) in the retina of the eye. Fluorescein dye is injected into a vein in the forearm. Over the span of an hour, it spreads through all the blood vessels and slowly leaks through the walls of the smallest. This leakage from retinal vessels causes the clear jellylike substance (vitreous humor) in front of the retina to glow when exposed to brief flashes of ultraviolet light. The amount of glow, which is measured electronically, is proportional to the amount of dye leakage. Abnormally high values are found after several months of poorly controlled diabetes and appear to correlate with glycosylated hemoglobin values.

R   Regular insulin; abbreviation used in this manual.

Receptor sites; receptors, insulin   Glycoprotein (glucose and protein) molecules, located on the outer surface membrane and internal membranes of cells, that bind insulin so that it can facilitate the transport of glucose across the particular membrane. Other hormones may bind to other receptor sites.

Regular insulin   A clear, rapid-acting insulin that exerts most of its biological effects within 4 hours after subcutaneous injection.

Renal   Relating to the kidney.

Retinopathy   Noninflammatory diseases of the retina. In poorly controlled diabetes, this takes the form of degeneration of the retinal blood vessels which show fluid leakage in early stages, and hemorrhages, etc., leading to possible blindness, in the late stages.

S   Semilente insulin; abbreviation used in this manual.

Saccharides   Carbohydrates, sugars.

Serum   The clear fluid that remains after clotted material has been removed from blood; blood—less blood cells and clotting factors.

Simple sugars   Monosaccharides and disaccharides: sugars consisting of only one or two molecular building blocks and therefore capable of being more rapidly digested than complex sugars. Examples include the monosaccharides glucose and fructose, and the disaccharides lactose, sucrose, and maltose.

Subcutaneous   Beneath the skin. The usual route of injection for exogenous insulin and glucagon.

Sucrose   Table sugar. A disaccharide of glucose and fructose.

Triglycerides   The principal type of fat stored by the body as reserve fuel. One of the risk factors for cardiovascular diseases. They can be manufactured in the liver from glucose with the result that serum triglyceride levels are usually elevated when BG is elevated. Fasting serum triglyceride levels were used as indicators of recent diabetic control prior to the availability of glycosylated hemoglobin measurements.

Type I diabetes   Insulin-dependent diabetes (IDDM). Usually caused by loss of function of most or all pancreatic B-cells. Patients in this group develop ketoacidosis if not treated with insulin.

Type Ia diabetes   The more severe subclass of Type I, where C-peptide levels are less than 5 percent of normal. Most juvenile-onset diabetics fall into this group. Also called brittle, labile, or severe diabetes.

Type Ib diabetes   The less severe subclass of Type I, where

C-peptide levels are greater than 5 percent of normal, indicating that 5–50 percent of pancreatic B-cells still remains.

Type II diabetes   Non-insulin-dependent diabetes (NID-DM). The milder forms of diabetes. Onset is usually after age 40.

Type IIa diabetes   Nonobese, non-insulin-dependent diabetes. A subclass of Type II.

Type IIb diabetes   Obese non-insulin-dependent diabetes. The subclass of Type II that includes 85 percent of diabetics. These patients are usually at least 20 percent overweight. Glucose intolerance is frequently caused by reduced availability of insulin receptor sites in insulin-dependent tissues, a condition that somehow accompanies obesity. Appropriate treatment is usually weight reduction.

UL   Ultralente insulin. A turbid, very long-acting insulin, without modifying proteins.

Venous blood   Blood removed from a vein (usually in the arm).

INDEX

A-cells, 38, 40
acetone, 40
Actenberg, J., 2n
adenosine triphosate (ATP), 195, 196
adolescence, 48, 119
  nonimmune resistance in, 56
adrenal hormones, 41–42
alanine, 114
albumin, 111
alcohol, 151, 154, 164, 166–167, 177
  undetected hypoglycemia and, 173–174
allergy, insulin, 116, 129
American Diabetes Association (ADA), 6, 145, 156n, 165, 166, 171–172, 216
American Heart Association, 145, 155
amino acids, 40, 41, 114, 149, 150, 154, 201
amputation, 1, 2
amylase, 147, 154
angiography, 13
aprotinin, 56
artificial sweeteners, 165–166
aspirins, 128, 178
atherosclerosis, 8

atrophy, 32
AUTOLET lancet holders, 67, 77, 79, 217
  use of, 84, 85–87

BAYg 5421, 169
B-cells, 38, 51–52, 53, 55n, 57
  biphasic response of, 39, 52
  catecholamines and, 41
  measurement of insulin produced by, 44, 47–48, 58, 59–60
bile acids, 168
Bio-Dynamics, 66, 67, 69, 77
Bio-Science Laboratories, 48
birth control pills, 125n, 129
birth defects, 45–46, 53
blindness, diabetes as cause of, 1, 2
blood, venous vs. arterial, 94
blood glucose (BG):
  in brittle or labile patients, 49, 50
  carbohydrate increase after stabilization of, 162–163
  conflicting views on control of, 5–7
  daily measurements of, 19, 21
  differences in lab and patient measurements of, 84, 94–95
  equipment for measuring of, 21, 66–83